The Foul Bowel

101 Ways to Survive and Thrive With Crohn's Disease

John Bradley
Illustrations by Rose Hutchings

The Foul Bowel: 101 Ways to Survive and Thrive With Crohn's Disease

Published in 2010 by Yknot Publishing, a division of Yknot Strategic Solutions Inc.

Visit our website at www.Foulbowel.com

Printed in the United States of America by Createspace, On-Demand Publishing Inc.

ISBN 13 digit: 978-0-9866200-0-3

ISBN 10 digit: 0986620009

To Martin
1955-2003

Acknowledgments

THIS IS THE first time I have shared anything but the bare details of my Crohn's saga beyond my immediate family. I am not alone in my reticence as it is a typical behavior of Crohn's patients. Because many of the symptoms are of a deeply personal and embarrassing nature, we tend to not broadcast the latest state of our bowels.

So a huge thank you to my dedicated readers of early drafts whose feedback helped me shape what began as a meandering personal account into something that could be of interest and help to not only Crohn's patients but anyone who knows someone with the disease and gets told as little about it as did my friends and relatives.

My wife Audrey, mother Margaret and brother Andrew have been the heart of my editorial committee, along with Lee Bate and Norma Boultwood. I am grateful to Jayne Tilt, Jennie McNeill, Christine Moulden, Jude Hindle and Sharon Boyce for providing valuable feedback on early drafts, and to Cheryl Coley-Smith, Madeleine Gunn and Steve Reiman for digging into their memory banks. Annie Dunseith opened my eyes to the world of self-publishing, Paula Costello did a sterling job copy editing the text and my daughter Georgina assisted in developing the website www.Foulbowel.com.

Lastly, an enormous thank you to a dear friend and work colleague, Rose Hutchings, for her marvelous illustrations and cover design which I feel really encapsulate the spirit of the book, and it is to her late husband and friend of mine, Martin Hutchings, that this book is dedicated.

Foreword

"It's no longer a question of staying healthy. It's a question of finding a sickness you like."

– Jackie Mason

HAVING CROHN'S DISEASE is like being transported back to being an infant. People talk at you using an incomprehensible language. No one seeks, welcomes or values your opinion. Mom, in the guise of the medical profession, most definitely knows what's best for you. Your food is bland, mushy and generally appalling. Your poop becomes an object of fascination for others. Consequently, it is not unusual for a Crohn's patient to feel as helpless as a two-year old.

But it does not need to be so. Through trial and error I have discovered that having Crohn's disease is something you can improve at if you approach it with the right attitude. As with any other aspect of life, when you're ill, it's to your advantage to try and be successful at it.

By that I don't mean heroically finding a cure (there is no cure for Crohn's), or fighting the illness every step of the way (those people tend to die young). Nor do I mean being a model patient, hanging on every word of wisdom imparted by the massed ranks of the medical profession (model patients tend to have the worst prognosis of all). What I do mean is that being successful at having Crohn's disease is about being able to take ownership for your illness and its treatment. The outcome is not just the feeling of triumphing over the medics – although that has its moments – but is about not letting your illness impact your enjoyment of life.

Over a seven-year period I had to see a lot of doctors and have my orifices endlessly probed before I was finally diagnosed at the age of 23 with Crohn's disease. Since then, I have spent almost thirty years dealing every day with illness, drugs, medics and the not-so-occasional surgery. But, by learning to see the funny side of the ridiculous medical procedures we undergo; by being reminded each and every day of the value of good supportive relationships with family, friends and colleagues; by realizing that Crohn's disease need not restrict the freedom we have to find our own path through life; by seeing that there are still opportunities to make good choices, the successfully ill have as happy and fulfilled a life as anyone else. This is true despite having an endless cycle of symptoms, surgeries and drug regimes that healthy people would find appalling to contemplate.

My thirty-year grappling match with the illness and the medical profession has taught me more than I would have ever thought possible about how to achieve this goal. In telling you my medical odyssey, I hope to share with you the insights, skills and tips I have picked up in not just surviving my Crohn's but thriving with it.

Tip #1: Take Your Pick

You have a choice how to be ill. You can attempt to carry on as though nothing is wrong and end up killing yourself in the process. Or you can be a victim, weeping and wailing "Why me?" at every turn and killing yourself spiritually in the process. Or you can be a Positive Acceptor: recognizing that your Crohn's is a card you have been dealt in the poker game of life, but one that will not take away your ability to play your hand to the full.

Table of Contents

Diagnosis Day

"Diagnosis: a preface to an autopsy"

– Anon

I SAT ALONE and seemingly forgotten in one of the closet-like consulting rooms of the gastro-intestinal clinic at Birmingham's Royal Free Hospital. Over the previous seven years I had sat in similar rooms countless times, only to have the medic stare at his notes while mumbling the profession's many different and obtuse versions of "Sorry buddy, we haven't a clue what's wrong with you". It is amazing how many ways they have of saying this, all the time sounding as though they do actually know what's going on. "We just need to run a few more tests to make sure", "I think things seem a little better so we'll keep going as we are", and so on ad infinitum. I strongly suspect there is a secret part of the Hippocratic Oath that commits a doctor to never owning up to being baffled.

Because of the medical profession's reluctance to acknowledge fallibility, I had, over the seven years up to that point, been subjected to an endless series of apparently random tests, followed by a variety of treatments for the latest wild guess as to the source of my increasingly dire problems. This hit-or-miss approach had eventually run out of options, only to be followed by the inevitable descent into it all being my fault – stress – then it being pinned on the last resort of the baffled doctor— depression. So I did not have a great sense of anticipation at being there once again.

Although these rooms are as bursting with sensory stimulation as an undertaker's parlor, I had by this time discovered ways of keeping myself amused while waiting to be graced by the presence of a doctor. I weighed myself on that intriguing example of pre-industrial technology where you move the little weights along the bar. One-hundred-and-thirty pounds: my lowest yet. However, the long ruler affixed to the wall reassured me that I was still 5' 8", so it was not all bad news.

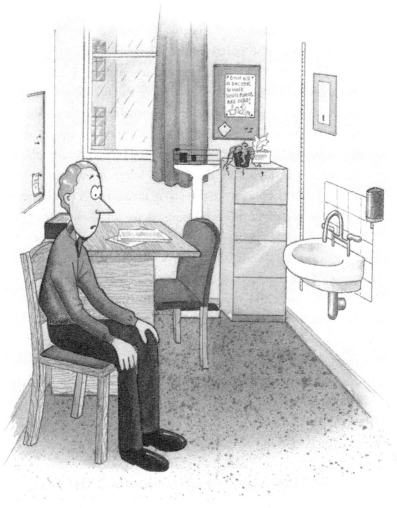

Waiting on a word

Then, of course, pinned to the otherwise barren notice board, was the ubiquitous medical cartoon snipped from one of the more venerable copies of Reader's Digest. This timeless classic was the "Don't use a doctor whose houseplants are dead" one, located above a very sad cactus that looked like it had endured a particularly dry summer in Death Valley. Do doctors find these cartoons funny? Do they think we will?

There was also a complete absence of reading material to pass the time. I don't know what hospital administrators get up to all day when there is so much scope for improvement. If the gastro-intestinal clinic managers had the good sense to procure the same reading matter as did their more enlightened counterparts in the infertility clinic (more on that later), hospital appointments would be a lot less soul-destroying and consequently good for business. But having said that, the gastro clinic was always jammed and running three hours late, so perhaps the management felt that subscriptions to Naughty Neighbors, Urban Nudist and Spankers Weekly would be difficult to justify.

I have come to the conclusion that we're forced to spend so much time waiting for doctors in these desolate rooms in order to break our spirits and make us more susceptible to agreeing with everything they say. After twenty-five minutes of staring blankly at the pale green painted wall, I have usually forgotten everything I planned to say to the doctor or sometimes why I'm there at all. Perhaps it's like this in Guantanamo Bay.

Tip #2 – Stay Alert

Do not be intimidated by the waiting process; feel free to amuse yourself any way you can while enduring the wait. If there's a stethoscope, listen to your own heartbeat. If

you're very lucky, you will find one of those special rubber hammers for testing your reflexes. If you're caught in
the act you will merely get a raised eyebrow, but at least
your brain will still be functioning.

Just as I was considering the possibility that I was in fact the last
man alive, the rest of Birmingham having been obliterated in some
kind of catastrophe, the door opened and in walked the senior
registrar of the gastro-intestinal surgical team. Amber alert: I was
seeing the second in command rather than the usual overseas
student. RED ALERT: He was not only making eye contact but had
a definite gleam of triumph as he broke it to me.

"Good news Mr. Bradley, we know what is wrong with you."

So staggered was I at hearing a definitive statement relating to
my condition that I almost missed the punch line.

"You have Crohn's disease!"

YEEEESSSSSSS!!!!!!! If this had been a football match, I would
have been cautioned for my ludicrously excessive touchdown
celebration. I may have ripped off my shirt and thrown it to the
massed drones in the main waiting room, I can't quite remember. At
last my worries were over! Surely the super-slick medical machine,
after the seven-year glitch in diagnosis, could now purr into action.
As my initial surge of euphoria passed, I realized he was still talking

"…and this hospital is one of the world's leading centers for the
treatment and management of Crohn's disease." I now felt guilty for
ever having doubted the medics. How lucky was I? World experts!
Lead me on!

In complete contrast to the glacial pace of events for the previous half-decade and more, he then jauntily snapped up the phone,
called the head of this world-renowned Crohn's disease facility, and
arranged for me to go straight up. You could stuff your six-month

waiting list up your rectum – I was on the fastest of fast tracks now! So off I went to the place that would become my second home for the next fifteen years - Ward 8 of the Birmingham Royal Free Hospital.

As I navigated the corridors, still euphoric that I had a known illness as opposed to a completely undetectable and imminently fatal condition, I began to ponder what lay ahead. Well, actually, at that precise moment, the urology ward lay ahead. Backtracking to find the obscured sign towards Ward 8, I had a jaunty step, not realizing how much every single aspect of my life was going to be impacted by the condition first documented by Dr. Burrill Bernard Crohn in 1932.

Well, it wasn't exactly all his own work. Burry, as I like to think of him, was one of three authors of a paper entitled "Regional Ileitis: A new clinical entity". His two colleagues, Dr. Leon Ginzberg and Dr. Gordon D. Oppenheimer, missed out on ever-lasting fame by dint of alphabetical order. Which is a shame really; telling people I had Oppenheimer's disease would have sounded so much better, conjuring up images of being at the cutting edge of science: "Yes, it all came from the NASA program along with Teflon and write-upside-down pens." I would have been a social magnet, something that is definitely not the case with Crohn's disease, which sounds like an affliction suffered by mad old women who keep herds of stray cats. Still, things could have been worse; the authors could have merged their names, calling it Croginzen-heimer's Ileitis, which would have sounded like some sort of mental illness.

Given that everlasting fame only devolves to the first named author of these team efforts, it is a surprise that more have not made use of the deed poll to change their names and leapfrog their way to the top. But then confusion would reign as we would only suffer from illnesses beginning with the letter "A", "Oh, you think I might have Aardvark's disease? I thought Aaron's malady was more likely, or perhaps Aasvogel's syndrome." But there are signs it may be happening: a quick internet search tells me there are at least 337 illnesses beginning with the letter "A", three times the number of illnesses that begin with the letters W,X,Y and Z combined. Now you know why.

As I approached the frosted glass doors that marked the boundary of Ward 8, I had no idea that it would be the source of much pain, misery, distress, frustration, anger, tears and clenching of teeth (and that would just be from listening to Hospital Radio). I pushed through the swing doors and enquired as to the whereabouts of the head honcho, a Dr. Ray. Having been directed to his office, I was struck by his cadaverous features and a booming voice so deep that blue whales plumbing the icy depths of the Barents Sea would have followed his half of the conversation. With white coat, firm handshake and multiple framed certificates on the wall, here, I thought, was my savior.

However, things did not get off to a good start for either of us.

"I'm not sure why he sent you up right now," rumbled the basso-profundo, which I more felt in my chest cavity than heard. A patient turning up out of the blue was clearly not a welcome sight. Doctors, I have discovered, do not cope well with spontaneity. They like to have complete control of proceedings. You seldom get the response you want when you spring surprises on them. Rather than employ the tactics of the leopard hunting gazelles on the Serengeti, you must think like the spider, coaxing your prey to where you want it, all the while giving it the impression that it, not you, is in charge.

Tip #3: Think Like a Spider

You should always pre-plan any encounter with a doctor. Know what you want from the appointment; have your facts rehearsed and at your fingertips; think how you will phrase things so that you still sound deferential. If you just turn up and start calling the shots, you will usually hit the brick wall of medical intransigence.

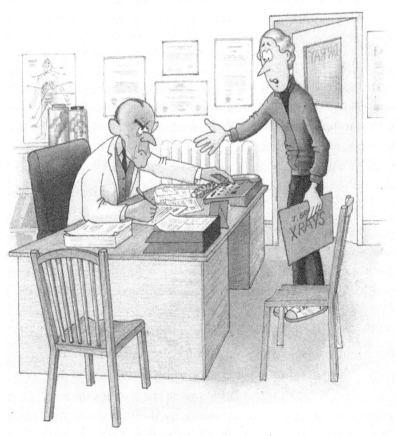

Dr. Ray, I presume?

Dr. Ray's vacillation somewhat deflated my euphoria, but his heart was not made of stone. Moved by my crestfallen expression, his hand, which had been poised to summon the heavy mob from the secretary's office, paused over the intercom button.

"Well you're here now. Let's have a look at the X-rays".

I perhaps should have mentioned that I had made the trek to Ward 8 clutching a very large envelope that contained the photographic evidence which had led to my diagnosis. A couple of weeks earlier, I had been subjected to a test known as a barium meal. This test, in which I now consider myself something of an expert having endured it another nine times over the years, is deceptively benign-sounding.

It begins two days prior to the main event with the instruction that one has to cease eating and restrict the diet to clear fluids. This means no milk and being only able to consume things like cups of tea or, as a special treat, jelly. As anyone who has undergone this regimen will tell you, there is no hunger like that which hits you after 24 hours of such abstinence. I would have eagerly snatched food from my starving grandmother's mouth. But soon this primal urge to eat anything or anyone pales into insignificance as you enter the bowel-clearing phase which is essential in order for clear pictures to be taken of your insides.

I have read that the ancient Romans enjoyed nothing more than a good purgative, though I fail to see the attraction myself. Drinking gallons of a salty solution to induce at least a dozen frenzied dashes to the john might have passed as entertainment when the barbarians were at the gates, but it leaves a lot to be desired in the digital era. The only way to get through the ordeal of passing gallons of what seems like sulphuric acid is to imagine the delicious foods upon which one will gorge once the whole event is over.

But there is another sting in the tail. After the barium meal itself you completely lose your appetite: the much anticipated juicy steak turns to ashes in your mouth. This is because of the process itself. One is forced to consume in rapid order a couple of pints of what initially seems like a strawberry milkshake. In fact the illusion continues until the very point of consumption. The orderly whips up the mixture with an electric whisk; it has the uniquely artificial color of a strawberry milkshake; it even smells like one. But the first gulp comes as a shock: it has the consistency and texture of wet cement.

A compound of the metal barium – barium sulphate - is required to act as a contrasting agent in the bowels, which then will show up clearly when bombarded by X-rays. Fair enough; bowel is soft tissue so would otherwise blend into the background. Barium's qualifications for this task can be gleaned from the origins of the word itself, deriving from the Greek word *bary*, which means "heavy". But while its heaviness is a benefit in being able to stop the passage of X-rays, there is a downside for the patient: barium sulphate is really, really heavy. The gloop has to be consumed quickly and in its entirety so that you have a big, solid mass of sludge going through your system. Otherwise you have to undergo the whole rigmarole again.

The icing on the cake to a procedure that would have led to much back-patting in the new product development laboratories of the Spanish Inquisition is that you get an injection designed to speed the progress of the barium through the bowel, which would otherwise take a day or three, depending on your own personal digestive system settings. The result being that your digestive tract goes into overdrive with much internal grumbling and sloshing to add to your discomfort.

Your troubles continue immediately after the x-raying is over as the barium drink, now mysteriously shorn of its strawberry coloring, comes racing through. The final indignity is that once the initial rush of liquid barium has passed, its residue seems to hang around forever, coating your doings with a ghostly hue that imparts the buoyancy of divers' boots. No amount of flushing or vigorous toilet brush thrusting can shift the evidence past the u-bend until one is forced to don the rubber gloves and solve the problem manually.

So although the entire event takes upwards of a week from beginning the starvation phase to one's bowels returning to normal, the meat and potatoes of the exercise is spending a mere half hour lying on a flat and extremely hard table being bombarded by five years' worth of radiation. To get better pictures, the radiologist uses a variety of implements to manipulate your bowel loops into the photographic frame. The only benefit is that usually, if you twist your head around, you can see what he is seeing on the screen. I must admit to finding that part fascinating; watching the graceful peristalsis of one's own bowels feels a bit like looking into one's soul.

Tip #4 – Get Smart

Although the X-ray monitor is set up for the convenience of the radiologists rather than for your optimal viewing, it is always a good idea to get as clear a look as you can. It's your body after all and knowledge gained now on what's going on inside can stand you in good stead when you're told the official results days or weeks later. However, don't pester the radiologists as they really do need to concentrate on what they're doing, but if they seem to be the chatty type, throw in the odd question about what you're seeing on the screen. If you're lucky, you will get a guided tour around your guts.

Back in Doctor Ray's office, it was the X-ray photographs, which he was putting up on his light-box, that contained all the evidence needed to confirm the presence of Crohn's disease. He pointed out three different areas where the small bowel, normally a good inch in diameter, seemed to have shrunk to no more than a tenth of that. These areas, called strictures, were a classic Crohn's symptom. What the image showed was not that the bowel had shrunk, but that it was, in fact, badly inflamed. When tissue inflames it expands and, as the bowel is a tube, that expansion had reduced the diameter of the tube to next to nothing. This, he explained, accounted for most of my symptoms.

While I found this bit of the impromptu consultation interesting, I was somewhat less enthralled by what followed. In addition to the findings from the barium meal, which were new news, he pointed out a series of other symptoms I was sporting that added up to, he proclaimed, a classic case of Crohn's disease. Firstly, I was malnourished: 130 lbs on a 5' 8" frame is skinny, really skinny. Added to that, I was massively anemic, which he demonstrated by asking me to outstretch my palm, which was undeniably a uniform white, even in the creases. Even the least perceptive fortune teller in the carnival would have had her easiest palm reading ever with me: "You are going to be very, very ill and very, very soon."

I also had a plethora of other indicators, the most shocking to me being that my fingers were clubbed, as in rounded rather than ending in a bit of a point. I had honestly never thought about the shape of my fingertips, nor that they might be different to anyone else's. But apparently they were, and still are. This is obvious to me today when I attempt to use a BlackBerry, my stumpy fingers being unable to straddle fewer than three keys simultaneously, rendering my messages completely incomprehensible.

So the bottom line was that, in Dr. Ray's opinion, this all added up to a textbook case of Crohn's disease. Which raised the question in my mind as to why, if it was so bleeding obvious, had diagnosis taken seven years from the onset of the first major symptom? It never takes that long on House, but then a TV show where no one gets diagnosed for the first seven seasons might not be a huge hit. I know it wasn't a huge hit with me.

Crossed Wires

"My illness is due to my doctor's insistence that I drink milk, a whitish fluid they force down helpless babies."
   – W.C. Fields

OF COURSE, the diagnosis was not the start of my medical odyssey. By that time I was a grizzled veteran of the system and had long since lost the innocent optimism with which we all approach our first encounter with a doctor, an optimism relentlessly created and nurtured by the most impressive PR operation the world has ever seen.

Throughout the last 50 years, we have all been subjected to a ceaseless barrage of good press for all things medical. And it continues today where every newspaper or magazine has weekly or even daily sections devoted to the expounding of a seemingly infinite number of medical breakthroughs. Yet the government can't build hospitals fast enough, so something doesn't add up.

But I went into the medical system as a firm believer, for two good reasons. Firstly, I had watched all the medical dramas and soaps of the 1960s and '70s, from Doctor Kildare to Marcus Welby M.D. via Dr.Quinn and Doogie Howser, where doctors were universally depicted as being omniscient. A few probing questions, a donning of the stethoscope and a tapping of the upper back as though searching for a stud behind drywall preceded the inevitably infallible pronouncement, all the while winking at the giggling nurses at the end of the bed.

The second reason I subscribed to Doctor Knows Best was that, when I was growing up, we had a cheerleader for doctors in our household. My mother spent her entire career in nursing, rising from being a ward nurse up to being the nursing training manager for our local health district, topped off with a couple of inventions of nurse training aids patented in her name. With such an advocate for the medical profession in the house, it was natural that I should concur, even though my one major medical encounter during my formative years contained a clue that perhaps all was not quite as it seemed.

When I was four years old, I was suffering from a discharge from both ears. This is the kind of condition that causes differing reactions in the school playground: revulsion in the girls, contrasted by admiring gasps of amazement from the boys. My mother, who at that time was the nurse in the outpatients department of the Blackburn Royal Infirmary, sided firmly with her gender and saw it as something to be sorted out ASAP. Consequently, she immediately took me to see the ear, nose and throat consultant – there's no point having a medical background in the family if you can't jump the queue.

As he peered into the back of my mouth, using a miners' lamp and a popsicle stick as implements, he breezily announced, "Well, you'll be a lot better off without those", which signaled the imminent demise of not just my adenoids – the most likely suspect – but my tonsils for good measure. Back then, you were lucky to survive any contact at all with the medical profession and emerge with your tonsils intact. Nowadays, the incidence of infants having their God-given tonsils forcibly removed has declined by 90%. Medical opinion seems to have caught up with common sense that they might be there for a reason.

In hindsight, what I should have said to the scalpel-happy hacker, despite running the risk of coming over as a somewhat precocious four-year-old, was, "I beg your pardon? Better off without those? Would you mind telling me why one of God, the Intelligent

Designer or a Selfish Gene would have put tonsils in there if it was better for all concerned that you whip them out the first time I have an affliction that raises my status in my peer group?" Of course I said no such thing and merely noisily celebrated the fact that I would be living off ice cream for the next week, my medical faith still intact.

Tip #5: Speak Up at the Back!

When a doctor announces a course of action, usually in a tone that conveys 100% certainty, the lifetime's worth of pro-medical PR with which you have been bombarded impels you to say, "OK". Always resist that urge. Any response, no matter how feeble, that queries the course of action is always better as it will force the doctor to explain a little more of his reasoning. Most times it will make no difference, but on the odd occasion it will give you information that you can take away to check out for yourself.

And that was the sum of my medical experience until what would eventually turn out to be Crohn's disease reared its flatulent head fourteen years later. Of course I contracted chicken pox, along with every other child in our village; but, somewhat mysteriously, I was spared the measles plague that cut a swathe through my social circle the next year. My elder brother Andrew succumbed, and, even though we shared a bedroom, I remained resolutely unblemished. No one could understand why I had been spared this pestilence. But, despite these common childhood ailments, the fact is that, for most who contract Crohn's disease, or any other major, chronic condition, it will be the first time we are sucked into the medical machine.

So I was basically a healthy child, growing up in the little village of Tockholes, which is about three miles south of Blackburn in England. I had all the benefits of fresh air, fields and woods to play in, and built up my young muscles every summer helping the local farmer bring in the hay bales. Country pursuits such as drinking water from springs that sprang down-field from herds of cows who liberally filled the water-table with their poop seemed to do me no harm. No doubt due to a more than robust immune system, my school photographs show me to be what I considered at the time rosy-cheeked. But, with the benefit of hindsight, I must confess to having been a touch chubby, despite my active lifestyle.

Having said that, my diet was not quite the same as everyone else's. Perhaps the biggest clue was that I did not like the fries that came with school lunches, whereas all my friends could have quite happily eaten nothing else. So great was my distaste for them that I would sometimes sell my lunch token to one of the older kids. It wasn't that I just didn't like fries, but if they were less than perfectly fresh, they turned to ashes in my mouth. In addition to my fries aversion, I had no time for vegetables, but this could still be considered fairly normal behavior for a teenager.

Less usual was an addiction I had had as long as I could remember, and had made no effort whatsoever to wean myself off: I just loved to sneak spoonfuls of granulated sugar when no one was looking. Even now, I cannot resist filching little sachets of sugar from restaurants. My idea of Nirvana is when there appears at the table a silver bowl containing sugar lumps, especially those irregularly-shaped, artisanal ones, which I consume as though in training to take on the part of Mr. Ed, the talking horse of the eponymous 1960s television show.

Here were the first two clues that Crohn's disease was on my horizon, although they went unnoticed at the time. Apparently,

Crohn's sufferers are statistically much more likely to eat more refined sugar and many fewer vegetables than average. No one yet knows if these are causes, symptoms or just irrelevant coincidences. It would have been harsh of me to be over-critical of the medical profession at this point for not having as yet come up with a diagnosis. After all, I hadn't told anyone about my food preferences – in fact, this is the first time I have ever confessed to selling my lunch tokens. Also, at that time in my life I wasn't feeling ill in the slightest.

Tip #6: Take an Interest

Without wishing to be an advocate of voluntary hypochondria, in hindsight I wish I had taken a bit more interest in the fact that my diet was different to those of every other single person I knew, and that I had told my mother about it. It's easy to get labeled a hypochondriac by busy doctors, but it's also easy to keep to yourself pertinent information because you either don't realize it might be significant or, even worse, because "you don't want to bother the doctor." If it's not normal, tell someone.

The first real clue that did register on my antennae happened during my first term away at university. At the age of 18, after completing High School, I had gone to the University of Manchester to study math and psychology. But the result was that, being so close to home - only twenty-five miles away – I returned to the nest most weekends to fulfill two objectives: get my clothes washing done and meet up with my girlfriend.

After a few of these trips, I did notice that those who knew me well were passing remarks along the lines that I must not be rising to the challenge of cooking my own meals, having observed that I was not quite as chubby-cheeked as when I had first gone away. As a first-year student, I was accommodated in a university hall of residence where one was expected to cook for oneself. There were hundreds of students in my particular hall with the arrangement of twelve single-sex bedrooms to a "dorm", each sharing a kitchen and bathroom.

I bitterly resented the accusation that I was failing to feed myself. I was having cereal for breakfast while many of my kitchenmates would just stagger bleary-eyed to the first lecture straight from having rolled out of bed. I usually had a cooked lunch at the university refectory, and was dishing up what I considered to be some quite wholesome and tasty dinners: steak, eggs over easy and piles of instant creamed potato being my favorite.

In fact, it was no mean achievement to be cooking any sort of meal at all in the circumstances. Having twelve young men share one four-ring electric oven would be difficult enough circumstances in which to shine gastronomically, but there were further challenges to contend with. Sharing one small fridge meant that much confusion arose as to who owned what in there, with the result that more often than not, one of your key ingredients would have gone AWOL at the critical moment. This shrinkage also extended to the dry and tinned ingredients. We each had a small locker, all secured by cheap padlocks, in which we stored our tins of beans and so on. However, we had in our midst a prolific and unrepentant thief who thought it perfectly reasonable to address his own shortages by picking a few locks until he found what he was after.

Even if you could keep your ingredients secure, the next challenge was in gaining adequate ring-time. Twelve hungry men, each cooking meals with two or three components, would put enormous strain on our kitchen's allocation of hot-rings and pots and pans.

This would get far, far worse when our kitchen's one Indian student, Raj, would invite what seemed like an entire caste of his chums round for a made-from-scratch curry. Not only did this tie up all four rings for hours on end, but the resulting caked-on curry that had splashed from the various bubbling cauldrons made the hob virtually unusable until someone chipped it off at the end of the week by which time the enamel had usually completely disappeared from sight.

But I was overcoming all these challenges. However, not only was I getting no credit for it, I was being roundly tut-tutted every weekend by the girlfriend, her mother and, of course, my mother, who all probably thought I was something of a mommy's-boy with no survival skills whatsoever. Each would try to outdo the other two in an arms race to fatten me back up again, but in vain. Although no one knew it at the time, I was gradually losing weight because Crohn's disease was reducing the effectiveness of my digestive tract. Indeed, the nearest to spotting it was a fellow kitchen user who could not help noticing that I was stuffing my face with mountains of fatten-you-ups brought from home, yet was clearly not gaining any weight. He would regularly ask me how my pet tape-worm was doing.

The false accusation concerning my ability to feed myself was my first encounter with what is usually the first major barrier you face to successfully being ill. When you are ill but are not yet aware of the fact, it seems that the default interpretation for an unclear set of symptoms is that you're not looking after yourself and therefore you are the cause of whatever symptoms ail you.

Tip #7 – It's Not Your Fault

There will be many instances where symptoms are airily dismissed or your diligence in sticking to a course of treat-

> ment is questioned. Do not bow to public opinion that you
> are the problem if you know that you are blameless – keep
> your self-belief.

So, although this early sign had perhaps been easy to fob off, the next one was to be a humdinger that was impossible to ignore, or blame me for, and would begin my thirty-year close encounter with doctors.

Now it is at this point in the book that I should perhaps run a warning advising readers that this story, through the necessity of describing the many wonderful symptoms of Crohn's disease, is not something you might want to be reading at the dinner table. As it is an illness that primarily affects the digestive tract, it should come as no surprise that many (though not all) of the symptoms in some way, shape or form, involve bodily functions and parts not normally brought up in conversation while taking tea with the vicar. So don't complain that you have not been warned.

The event in question occurred as I was contemplating the sports pages while clearing the traffic on the Hershey Highway. Yes, I was taking a dump. All seemed normal until, as I was finishing up and glanced downwards as my hand reached for the flush, I was stunned to see that the tissue in the bowl was completely bright red.

It seemed like every neuron in my body fired off simultaneously. I had never, in my entire life, had cause to be so disturbed by what confronted me in the bowl at the moment of flushing. If it had been just a smear, I'm sure I would have rationalized it as just a case of being a tad over-vigorous in the cleansing department, but there was no explaining this one away. It looked like a flimsy bandage just removed from a fresh shotgun wound.

Thinking that I was about to suffer the ignominious fate of bleeding to death while locked in with the Great White Throne, I dropped my trousers faster than a bishop in a brothel, grabbed handfuls of bathroom tissue and went to stem the flood. Only there was no flood. Surely, I thought, gaping wounds don't clot in a matter of seconds, but apparently mine had. However, the welcome relief of not having to deal with the unimaginable logistics of summoning help for a hemorrhaging rectum did little to mitigate the initial shock.

The next weekend I described this electrifying event to my mother, who then immediately booked me in to the family doctor for him "to have a look-see." A few days later, I assumed what would become, over the next thirty-two years, a wearisomely familiar position on the doctor's examining table as the first of many medical digits would attempt diagnosis by Braille. Lo and behold, the rectal groping did in fact discover the presence of some small hemorrhoids, so I was duly booked in to have an operation for their removal.

While I was delighted that something was being done, of course this would turn out to be a red herring. I had not been misdiagnosed as such – I did have a couple of hemorrhoids – but the problem was that, of Crohn's disease and hemorrhoids, the latter was assumed to account for a symptom that was in fact caused by the former.

There were two factors at play that combined to cause this misattribution. Firstly, I had only described a condensed version of my toilet trauma: motion, blood. I neglected to describe the fact that plenty of blood was followed almost immediately by hardly any blood at all. If it had been the result of piles, and quite small ones apparently, the initial quantity would have been less and the tailing off not so sudden. The reality was that I had not bled after passing a motion, but that I had passed a rather large and discrete quantity of blood, which is something entirely different. So I had not actually described an accurate version of events.

This was compounded by the second factor, which is what I consider to be the single most misleading bit of training given to doctors. To help allegedly very bright medical students grasp the self-evident fact that common illnesses are more common than rare ones, they have had drummed into them the phrase, "When you hear hoof-beats, think horses not zebras." But, in my experience, this invariably leads to the default assumption that all hoof-beats are caused by horses. In my case, because piles were present, they must be the cause of the bleeding.

The first question the doctor asked was designed solely to validate the initial hoof-beats of hemorrhoids, and was a very difficult question to answer anyway: "Did I strain?" Well, I don't know really. With intimate matters such as these, one has no other reference points as to what constitutes normal. How do you know what goes on in other people's boudoirs and water-closets? One man's straining is another man's gentle coaxing. So I umm'ed and ahh'ed to this question, which served only to convince the medic that I must have been having an eyeball-popping, almost heart-attack inducing battle of wills with the previous day's helping of curry-flavored instant potato. This had clearly, in the doctor's eyes, ruptured the piles – so problem solved. Now, of course, it is clear that in fact the piles were coincidental and whatever had occurred had been further upstream, where demons lurk.

The reason I so dislike the hoof-beats phrase is that, by its brevity and clarity, it negates the importance of context. I do agree that, on average, the hearing of hoof-beats would indicate the presence of galloping horses in the vicinity.

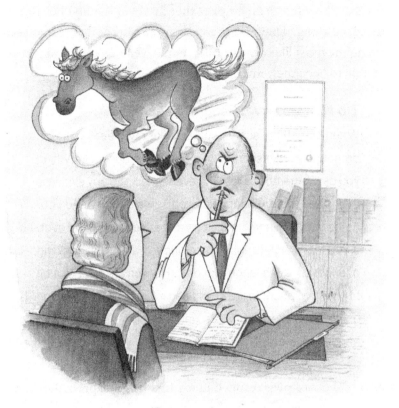

First past the post

But context and detail are everything. "Where were you when you heard hoof-beats?" is a question that could completely change the answer. The response, "Louisville racecourse on Kentucky Derby Day" would indeed strongly suggest the presence of horses. If, however, the answer was, "On the sweeping, majestic plains of the Serengeti", zebras or perhaps wildebeest would be worth a bet. See what I mean?

In order to be correctly diagnosed and avoid being trampled by hoof-beats, the small details are really important. Most doctors, in my experience, do not probe much beyond your own description of events, so, if that is incomplete they just hear the first hoof-beats that come along. They will then ask you a question aimed at confirming the most likely cause, but it could well be a question you are not able to accurately answer.

Tip #8 – Observe, Record, Describe

When something scary happens, like my bleeding, firstly, do not panic. As soon as you can, write down everything you can remember about the event and keep any evidence that is keepable. Then, when you see a doctor, read your notes out in full and bring along a spare copy to hand over. If you feel a significant point, or indeed any point, is being overlooked – challenge him on it. He won't like it, but a bit of an atmosphere in the consulting room is a lot better than going another seven years undiagnosed, which is what happened to me.

The discovery of piles resulted in my first hospital procedure since the premature termination of my tonsils, only this time there was not the prospect of an ice-cream diet to look forward to. The reward in this case was to be several days sitting on an inflatable ring, which still might have been appealing to a four-year-old, but at eighteen and with university lectures to attend alongside two hundred of my peers, I was less than enthused.

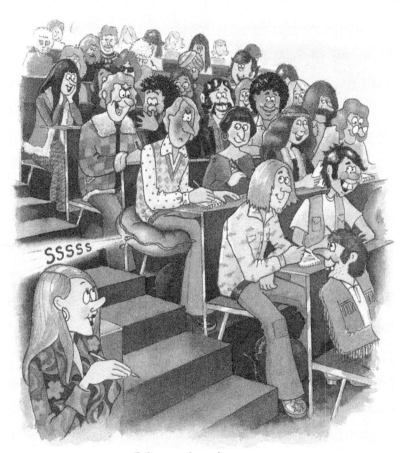

Piling on the embarrassment

Carry On Up The Khyber

"World's got two kinds of folks: them's that got piles and them that's gonna git 'em"

– Mrs. Manson in 'The Ladykillers', 2004

GOING INTO A HOSPITAL as a young adult is a very different experience to doing so as a small child, where a gaily decorated children's ward and the opportunity to make new, albeit temporary, friends make up for the trauma of the unknown. As a grown-up, you are much more aware of the depersonalizing and potentially embarrassing nature of the whole process.

The first stage of the prolonged humiliation is when you are sent to a spartan changing cubicle clutching a brace of hospital gowns. As you unfold these heavily starched, yet worryingly stained garments, the instructions to put this one on at the front and that one at the back seem to make little sense, as they appear to be identical. What if they are subtly different and you get them the wrong way round? Of course, no patient ever comes out from the cubicle to seek clarification. You are on your own now. A fact that becomes more apparent when you try to fasten the ties behind your back as they seem to develop a life of their own, playfully eluding your blind grasps.

There is little in life to match the feeling of vulnerability as you gingerly step out of your changing cubicle, wearing only two voluminous yet still flimsy gowns and a pair of disposable paper slippers. The initial worry as to whether or not you tied the right bits of string together pales into insignificance as you enter the public domain feeling more naked than you have ever done before.

The first thing you notice is that it is quite chilly, especially as, most likely, you are not used to cool air wafting freely in your nether regions. Then you are immediately propelled into the presence of other, equally discomforted people wearing exactly the same outfit. As with any visit to a hospital, plenty of waiting around is the order of the day. Of course, wearing next to nothing in the presence of complete strangers dampens down your desire to be sociable, so this initial waiting stage is inevitably conducted in a monastic silence and completely excludes even a glimpse of eye contact.

So, once again, any reading material whatsoever assumes a profound and deep level of interest as you pretend to be engrossed in an eight-year-old, extremely dog-eared Reader's Digest. You ignore the fact that half the pages are missing and the other half fall onto the floor with regularity.

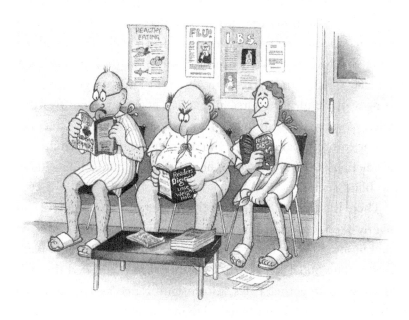

Relaxing in the waiting area

Your equally uncommunicative fellow travelers are picked off one by one as their names are called out from a sheet, and you soon begin to doubt that your name will ever be called at all. Have they forgotten you? Are you in the right waiting area, or even the right hospital? Again, no one ever lets his doubts turn into action as the uncalled sit there mute and forlorn.

You are also acutely aware that, due to the gown arrangement, your baby maker could be in full view of the people sat opposite, which prompts you to adopt the most convoluted seating position to exclude any possibility of exposure. One moment of inattention could result in you unthinkingly adopting the habitual male position of maximum angle between the legs or, even worse, crossing your legs. So the need for complete focus on the seating position means that you have no chance whatsoever of taking in a word on the page in front of you, or even of spotting that the pages you have open were reinserted upside down by a previous reader.

Finally, you are called through. But it proves to be the usual false dawn as you go round a corner only to see that your relatively cozy waiting area has been replaced by a handful of hard-backed chairs in a corridor. I'm sure Walt Disney learned his techniques of how to disguise the length of the wait from a past hospital visit; although he improved on the science with the idea that being entertained by Mickey Mouse enhances the passage of time better than staring at lime-green walls.

Tip #9: Take Something to Read

I have never once regretted taking something to read with me on a hospital visit. These places seem to operate in a parallel universe where time moves at one-tenth the speed it does outside. I sometimes buy small, inexpensive paperback editions of the classics just for this purpose. Sherlock

Holmes, Dracula, Dr. Jekyll and Mr. Hyde (not sure about that one), Treasure Island have all earned their cover price in keeping my mind off things while waiting around in hospitals.

Sitting in the corridor, you then experience another prolonged and unexplained wait, but this time without a randomly ordered Reader's Digest to capture your attention. You might be given a form to fill in or you may just sit there with only your potential groin visibility to keep you occupied. It is at this stage that worries creep in, no matter how outlandish. What if it goes wrong? How long will you be under the anesthetic? Will it be the Nitrous Oxide, last experienced in a nightmarish visit to the dentist's?

While the initial waiting area was mostly nurse-free, you are now in their territory and they are buzzing around like worker bees. And it is at this point you first experience every man's medical nightmare: the fear of the inappropriate and unjustifiable erection.

Of course, it makes no sense in the cold light of day; you cannot imagine a less erotic setting or occasion, which makes the fear ten times worse because there would be simply no way to explain it away. It is not that one thinks it likely that man's best friend will randomly spring into life; it is the certainty of the absolute humiliation that would follow should the unthinkable happen. There would be no hiding it. No number of gyrations could disguise the tent-like structure that the gowns would surely adopt. One might as well set off the fire alarm for the attention that would inevitably follow.

Alas, I have no advice to offer on dealing with this problem. In fact, I have found that the fear only worsens as you get older. At the age of 18, there is at least a shred of justification as the one-eyed beast does have a mind of its own. But at 50, I would just be a dirty old man. Even though it has never happened to me, the fear remains as gripping as it ever did. As the equipment ages and the chances of a random stiffy fade, the stakes get higher because the humiliation would be even deeper. I don't know what women worry about at this stage, perhaps they sit there thinking, "Oh my God! Is that dirty old man just pretending to read that upside down Reader's Digest while trying to look up my gowns? And I hope that fold in his gown isn't an ERECTION!!!"

Or maybe it's just me that has erection fear. After all, I have never discussed this issue with a fellow patient. Perhaps I was scarred by the fact that, as I waited in the corridor for the next stage of the pre-pile removal process, the nurse who approached me calling my name was someone I vaguely knew. She had been a classmate of my cousin, and I had briefly met and chatted to her at some school disco or other. Plus, she was nice-looking – in fact, a real hottie.

Uuuurrggh!!!! The potential embarrassment stakes had now shot into the stratosphere. Firstly, I probably had past form in having an erection while talking to this delightful girl. But much worse, not only would I have to face humiliation in some corridor of Blackburn Royal Infirmary, but that same humiliation could be broadcast to a social circle – my cousin's pals – who I considered to be my primary source of potential girlfriends should my current arrangements be terminated. I briefly considered if I would be protected by some kind of nurse-patient confidentiality clause, but rejected that as unlikely. So, with a complete and utter focus on completing difficult mental arithmetic sums, I followed her into the next stage of the process, enraged at myself for not being able to look away from her sashaying, pert-looking tushy.

Tip #10: Don't Ogle the Medical Staff

No good will come of it. Firstly, if you are male, why increase the risks of your own humiliating version of Barnum & Bailey's circus tent, and secondly, none of us look our best wearing institutional gowns so you will only be viewed as being sad and pathetic. If you forgot your book, close your eyes and go to your happy place (not THAT happy place, obviously).

Once I got into the inner sanctum, events sped up considerably. Before I could take in my surroundings, I was on a gurney with a drip in my arm. Then a reassuringly grey-haired anesthetist loomed over me, told me to count to ten in my head, and then I plunged into oblivion. I have tried many times to get to ten, but always failed. I felt a cold sensation in my arm as the anesthetic was pumped into my vein, then I was momentarily aware of a creeping wooziness before all was black.

Coming round from the anesthetic, as I became aware that I was in a bed in a room, who should be there but my nurse acquaintance? She brightly informed me that the procedure had gone well; two small hemorrhoids had been located and zapped, and that all looked well. She then slipped from nurse mode into acquaintance mode and blushingly informed me that, as she was wheeling me from the procedure room to where I now lay, my gowns had been bunched around my armpits until she had protected my modesty via a quick sartorial adjustment. She then admitted to being sorely tempted to tie a little ribbon around Charlie as a nice waking-up present for me, this apparently being a popular gag in the nursing sorority. I thanked her for sparing me this final humiliation that would no doubt have been embarrassingly broadcast to my girl-friend pool during some drunken binge.

Later that day, I was given my release papers and off I went, confident of not seeing the inside of a hospital for a lifetime. After the requisite couple of days sat on the rubber ring, all seemed well. In the following weeks, I had no more bouts of bloodletting and it seemed like the problem had been solved. Assuming that piles had been the problem, and no doubt caused by constipation, my girlfriend took it upon herself to send me off to Manchester on Sunday nights with a cake made, from what I could tell, entirely of All-Bran. The after-effects were as you would imagine, but in the interests of fending off any more hemorrhoid Hammer Horror moments in the lavatory, I meekly complied.

But the underlying problem hadn't been solved. My addiction to sugar lumps and antipathy towards vegetables and less than perfect chips continued unabated as mute evidence that Crohn's disease was still there, hidden from medical attention. More clues were to appear and fail to trigger a diagnosis. The next sign was a tendency towards mouth ulcers. This again is associated with Crohn's but I assumed was a more tangible sign that perhaps my diet still left a bit to be desired, so I failed to pass on the information.

The rest of my university years passed uneventfully in medical terms, which now makes me think that the illness must have spontaneously gone into remission. This again is a feature of Crohn's disease that presents a challenge to its diagnosis. It comes and goes completely unpredictably. Actually, it would be more accurate to say that the symptoms come and go; the disease itself never goes away.

Medical science, despite its many advances and its unceasing PR campaign, to me falls at the first hurdle with its inability to explain the feature of remission. I have not once heard a good explanation for why symptoms can disappear for months or even years, only to reappear later. We would not accept this apparent lack of understanding of the basic mechanics of a problem from any other profession. Would you trust a plumber who cannot explain why one day your tap drips profusely but then is perfect for a week before recommencing dripping again? Or an electrician who cannot explain why some days your house has power and other days not? But by giving this huge gap in knowledge a name – remission – doctors are able to maintain the impression of actually knowing what is going on.

Always get straight in your head in the most basic terms what is actually happening to you. Every medical event, especially surgery, is much easier to deal with once you have stripped away the gobbledy-gook because you can actually relate to what is going on. For example, a common surgery for Crohn's is to remove an affected part of the small bowel and then join up the ends of what's left. This is no different in principle to how a plumber fixes a burst pipe, yet surgeons refer to this most basic concept as a resection and anastamosis. It's as though they don't want us to know just how basic most surgery actually is.

Tip #11: Learn the Language

Every time you hear a medical term you do not understand, make a note of it and go and look it up. Also, when you are in with a doctor, do not hesitate to seek clarification by repeating back to her what she has just said with the rider, 'does that mean....', filling in the blank with your own understanding, but in plain English.

So, while in remission, my life returned to the normality of never thinking about illness, symptoms, doctors or hospitals. After graduating in 1979, I secured a job with Cadbury Bros., the chocolate firm, based at their centre of operations in Birmingham. My degree in math and psychology made, in my view, the ideal preparation for a career in market research, which was the position I had applied for in every company I could find that was looking to recruit graduates in that field. As luck would have it, towards the end of the recruitment process, my best opportunities had come with final interviews at Cadbury and Mars, and being held on reserve for a final interview at Rowntree. So it seemed that chocolate was going to be my calling.

Joining Cadbury would be one of the pivotal moments of my life. I would spend 24 years working for them; meet my future wife on my first day in the office, and benefit enormously from their enlightened and humane approach to helping employees cope with major illness. So, in September 1979 I relocated to Birmingham to begin my career.

Although I was immersed in getting to grips with my new job during the week, at weekends I dutifully traipsed back up to Blackburn to feed my decreasingly torrid love affair with my long-time girlfriend. It was during the last reel of this faltering romantic liaison that the Crohn's would awaken from its slumber and hit me with its next punch. By this time I had spent my hard-earned early pay slips on a battered old car, so was now driving up and down the highway. At the tail-end of a normal weekend, I would have my evening meal at my girlfriend's house then set off on the two-hour drive to Birmingham.

Somewhat mysteriously to me, this drive would be punctuated at some point by an agonizing stomach ache that would come from nowhere, last for around a minute and then disappear. And when I say stomach ache, this was not the gentle rumblings of overindulgence, but a doubling-up, sweaty forehead, breathless kind of pain –

not something that can be taken easily in one's stride while doing 85mph in the fast lane.

I had no idea what could be the cause of this agony. By then, the All-Bran cakes had long since been consigned to history as our relationship had become increasingly perfunctory, so I couldn't blame those. It was a complete mystery. So, once again, I passed it off as "one of those things" and didn't even mention it to my mother, let alone go to the trouble of finding a family doctor in Birmingham. It merely took its place alongside the sugar bingeing, vegetable avoidance, and grimacing as a sharp corner of a potato chip speared into the by now ubiquitous mouth ulcer, as unexplained aspects of my life.

I would finally be prompted into action one day in spring 1981. I had by then moved on from my first job at Cadbury in market research, and had taken a position in the marketing department as Assistant Brand Manager. One day, a new person had joined the Cadbury team at one of our advertising agencies and, as part of his education, had come to the factory for a tour on which I and my boss would accompany him, passing along various insights and facts as the tour progressed.

I was feeling absolutely fine until, it seemed, in an instant I was gripped by a stomach pain that dwarfed the highway variety. I could barely speak or walk, but gamely soldiered on, not wanting to disrupt this tour that had taken forever to arrange and for which the guy had come all the way from London. I had never felt time pass as slowly as it did then. The Cadbury factory site is colossal, so a tour in those days was a three-hour event. This was easily the longest three hours of my life to date. The pain, far from passing after a minute or so, would ebb and flow, each time coming back even more intensely. It was akin to enduring a very difficult childbirth while attempting to conceal the fact that it was even taking place.

Eventually I was able to deposit the visitor at the front door and tell my boss that I was going to have to go home. He expressed no surprise at all, saying that he thought I had looked dreadful on the tour, but had put it down to perhaps me having been on an absolute bender the night before. Having spent the evening quietly watching The Rockford Files, this seemed an unlikely explanation. So I dragged myself home and then, much to my surprise, immediately fell into a deep sleep despite the pain. Even more to my surprise, I awoke around an hour later feeling perfectly fine. Having by now found myself a family doctor, I booked myself in and was there a couple of days later, explaining this whole strange episode.

The doctor quizzed me on the nature of this pain, asking its location and if it was a sharp pain, a colicky pain and so on. Now one thing that all people who are chronically sick say is that it's a good thing you don't remember pain. However, in this case, it was a very bad thing. I couldn't recall the exact site; it seemed to fill my entire abdominal cavity, although I did seem to recall that it was even more intense in the upper part. Nor could I be of any help in describing its nature. How are you supposed to know what is a colicky pain and what isn't? More medical mumbo-jumbo and hoof-beat searching.

Doctors should know that pain is very difficult to describe, and should have developed a vocabulary that we patients can understand and use to describe it much more clearly. But they haven't. So he did the most logical thing for someone complaining of an unex-plained bout of stomach ache and booked me in for my next hospital visit to have my stomach examined visually.

What had actually happened, although I only post-rationalized this after my eventual diagnosis two years later, was that I had been stricken by the next major manifestation of my Crohn's disease. As I previously explained, an inflamed bowel lessens in diameter quite dramatically; so much so that improperly chewed food can get stuck. The bowel senses the blockage and attempts to clear it through spasms, and it is these that cause the pain.

On my highway trips, I had clearly been rushing my girlfriend's mother's meal and not chewing it properly, with the resulting pain a few hours later as I was Birmingham-bound. This time, though, I must have swallowed a really big piece of food – apple would be my best guess much later as this sequence of events was finally explained – and the spasms had not been able to clear it until the stomach acids and bile had gradually broken it down to the point where it must have finally disintegrated as I slept.

But none of this was apparent from my vague answers to the doctor's perfunctory tunnel-vision questions, so I unquestioningly complied with the prescribed action which was to undergo a process of internal eyeballing of the stomach known as an endoscopy, where a fiber-optic tube is pushed down your throat while you are under a mild sedation. In my case, I was out like a light and remember nothing of the event itself. But the aftermath was to trump the piles incident in terms of being another spurious diagnosis.

For a while, I had been in the habit of mixing myself a gin and tonic in the evening which may have contributed to a slight bout of acid reflux. The endoscopy had shown some mild irritation of my esophagus near the junction with my stomach. This was then automatically assumed to be the cause of the recurrent Sunday pain and the crippling episode in the factory. So I was told to avoid all alcohol for a while, stock up on the antacids, and be on my way.

Once again, the most common explanation was being sought, with questions thereafter only aimed at bolstering the initial diagnosis. Cowed by the white coats and general gravitas of the doctors passing such pronouncements, I meekly went along with their blithe assertions that a nightly gin and tonic could cause regular excruciating pain and the occasional three hours of almost unbearable agony. If this was the case, millions of people should have been similarly afflicted; national sales of gin would have gone through the floor, and the makers of Gaviscon and Tums become bigger than Exxon Mobil.

Tip #12: The Common Sense Test

Do not accept a diagnosis if it doesn't feel right to you or doesn't pass the common sense test. Many doctors latch onto a quick-and-easy diagnosis like a drowning man does a lifebelt. It's not as though we haven't been warned; this scenario is played out in every episode of House where people just shout out diagnoses off the top of their heads and the poor patient is taken to death's door by a succession of incorrect treatments. If challenging the medic gets you nowhere, ask to be referred elsewhere for a second opinion.

Alas, I was to be a victim of the superficial diagnosis for a third time as I returned a few months later to the family doctor complaining of yet more excruciating stomach pains. "What do you do for a living?" enquired the medic. My reply of "marketing" gave him a free hit. "Stressful is it?" Here was another of those leading questions where you have no reference points by which to calibrate your answer. "Well, I don't know really. Compared to being a postman or a librarian, I suppose it might be." And you can fill in the rest yourself. I got a lecture on the alleged benefits of reducing the stress in my life. Here was another incorrect diagnosis made on the flimsiest of evidence that delayed events even further.

Tip #13: Get Stressed about Stress

When you find yourself on the receiving end of a doctoral lecture on stress reduction in place of some real treatment or further investigation, it should immediately move you into red alert status. Quiz the medic hard on why he is doing this. Does it mean he has ruled out anything tangible? On what basis? Don't be shy, make him earn his corn in this situation; it can add months or years to your being eventually treated if you fall for the placebo treatment trick.

My eventual diagnosis that led me to Ward 8 would depend, not on a long-awaited flash of medical insight, but on happenstance. Two completely separate events would combine to finally make a diagnosis possible: I would become so ill that the fact I was actually ill finally became obvious even to the most hopeless student to scrape through medical school, and, through sheer chance, I would finally be seeing people with a modicum of expertise in Crohn's.

Darkest Before The dawn

"Without fear and illness, I could never have accomplished all I have."

— **Edvard Munch (Norwegian painter, 1863 - 1944)**

IT HAS SINCE been explained to me by an unusually candid gastroenterologist that the best thing a doctor can do when he doesn't have a clue what is wrong with you is to do nothing. Fair enough; the Hippocratic Oath they all take when rolling up the trouser leg does indeed bid them to "do no harm". But doctors who did nothing every time they were baffled would have the productivity of Homer Simpson. They would then be drummed out of the medical profession for giving the game away as to just how often their omnipotence is in fact mere impotence. So they have a beautifully crafted fall-back plan that not only masks their ignorance but actually reinforces the illusion that they always know what they are doing.

To keep the patient in mute subservience, they do nothing while appearing to be very confidently doing something, such as prescribing some placebo antibiotic or passing on advice about reducing stress. What then happens is that either the illness will clear up of its own accord, or failing that, will become so much worse that the increasingly obvious symptoms will trigger a light bulb in the medic's brain and recall a long-forgotten lecture last heard decades ago. In both cases, the doctor will get the credit for the cure.

I have to bow to such a brilliant deception, not least because I had been suckered into the charade of medical infallibility. Having first been given the "news" that the inflamed esophagus was the problem, I obediently adjusted my lifestyle to reduce, if not exclude, any and all possible food and beverage items that might be the source of the irritation, even though I had the appetite of a dieting gnat and a physique that would have prompted Gandhi to reach for the cream cakes. Because of a rogue diagnosis, the last remaining pleasures in my diet had now been snatched from my lips. Needless to say, this medically advised abstinence made no difference whatsoever to my condition other than to accelerate my weight loss. I had also taken the spurious stress message to heart and consciously cut back my working hours to no benefit whatsoever.

So why is it that I had been victim to yet another flawed diagnosis and pointless treatment regimen? First it was piles, then inflamed esophagus, then stress. Had I just been unfortunate in seeing the more hopeless members of the medical profession? I believe not, because this happens all the time. There were, I believe, two factors at play: I wasn't pushing back enough, and I was playing into their hands by only complaining about one thing at a time.

Now I know better, I would vigorously enquire as to how usual it is for two small piles to cause a major and unusual hemorrhage. I would get the doctor in a headlock until he admitted that mild irritation of the esophagus would not usually cause an otherwise healthy young adult to become completely incapacitated by pain. And, most of all, I would reject outright any diagnosis that contained the words "stress" and its bedfellow, "depression". Both just mean that no one knows what's wrong with you.

Tip #14: Push Back

Do not assume that you cannot contribute to the process of diagnosis. Ask the common-sense questions. Don't be afraid to interrupt their flow or to ask them to explain in layman's terms exactly what they are twittering on about. The best phrase you can use in these circumstances is, "Is

it normal to…" Your goal is to test the quality of their thinking and hopefully break through one-track-mind tunnel vision.

By only bringing up one symptom at a time, I was a victim to what I
call the Separate Hoof-beats Syndrome. The blood-letting and now
the stomach cramps had been investigated and, in both cases, some
very circumstantial evidence had been found to support the most
obvious diagnosis for each symptom. Each was then treated in
isolation.

Unfortunately, Crohn's disease manifests itself via multiple
symptoms where, for each, your real problem lies well down the list
of possible causes, so if you only bring up one of these at a time,
you then suffer a prolonged wait for the real answer. Far from being
an isolated glitch, it is in fact an inevitable outcome. Doctors have a
tendency to focus on the new news and seek only to treat the
specific problem you have come in about; they simply don't take the
time to reconsider your past medical history and see if there is a
deeper pattern emerging.

Actually, to be fair, they don't have the time to do the research
themselves. If they took half an hour to go over your entire medical
history and look to see a pattern emerging, that would give them
two problems. Firstly, their clinic would seize up completely as they
would have to do it for everyone. Joseph Stalin is quoted as saying
that "One death is a tragedy, a million deaths is a statistic." The
Health Department could equally well say that, "One ill person is a
medical problem, a million ill people is a logistical nightmare." So, in
dealing with the logistical problem of too many patients and too
little time, consultations are kept short – too short to do a full
medical history or much brain-racking looking for connections.

Tip #15: Run Down the Clock

Don't waste one second of the precious few minutes of your consultation chit-chatting about the weather. The clock is ticking in the medic's head from the second you walk in, so get to the point. Find out in your jurisdiction what the target consultation time is. Where I now live in Ontario, it is 14 minutes whereas I believe in the U.K. it is only 10 minutes. Americans have the advantage of paying for their doctor's time, so consultations tend not to be arbitrarily cut short. In all instances though, plan in advance to fit into whatever time you have a full summary of your past medical events and asking could there be any connection; are they related? Back up your questions with internet research beforehand: "I've read that...." They won't like it but they will be reluctant to kick you out if you are still within your time limit. And don't be ushered out early just because the clinic is running late.

I did eventually manage to benefit from this hopeless diagnostic charade due to the fact that I took the stress reduction message to heart in the workplace, not just in terms of my hours, but in my role. My early career as a brand manager in the marketing department had not got off to the greatest of starts. One of the problems was that apparently I had little credibility with the sales force whose job it was to sell the various new lines and marketing promotions that were supposed to be my output. Naturally, I was very stressed to hear this and resolved to put things right, as stress reduction was now a major goal in life.

Establishing personal credibility is a tricky issue in the business world, especially with hard-bitten salesmen. I soon determined that the only sure-fire way to get them onside with Team Bradley would be for me to successfully have carried the sales bag. Other brand managers who had joined the marketing department straight from university had to spend their first six months with the company out on the road working as salespeople. Because I had joined another function, I had missed out on this grounding. So I went back to my boss and put in a request to spend a few months on the sales force. My application was rubber-stamped and my name put down for the next sales training course, which Cadbury ran three or four times a year at their Management Training College.

But while knowing the salesman's key tricks would stand me in good stead throughout life, the main benefit of the course for my eventual diagnosis was in what came afterwards, in that a life on the road precipitated a dramatic decline in my health. Not that this would be a benefit in itself as I would be exceptionally ill for months, but there is no doubt that it did facilitate my eventual diagnosis.

During my nine-month stint as a salesman, I had three postings to parts of the country, ending in a spell in deepest west Wales. The company was generous in its allowances, meaning that I was staying in decent hotels during the week. I had a company car, expense account and what would be, for me, a completely wasted chance to eat gargantuan hotel meals. This golden opportunity to pile on the pounds was going to waste as I felt increasingly off my feed due to the Crohn's getting insidiously more severe.

In each of the hotels, I had struck up nodding relationships with other lost souls who were in the same boat of being away from home during the week. In Swansea I would usually dine with a Cardiff-based bank manager who was covering for his sick Swansea counterpart. Consequently, I had a barometer against which I could compare food habits, and it became apparent to me that my appetite was by now appalling and clearly worsening by the week.

As we took our seats in the dining room, my ears would be assailed by the sounds of lips being smacked and belt buckles being loosened while I gazed glumly at the gravy-stained menu of the day. When I thought I was full, which invariably happened with at least half of the serving still on my plate, my co-diners would be guzzling on as though aware of an impending famine.

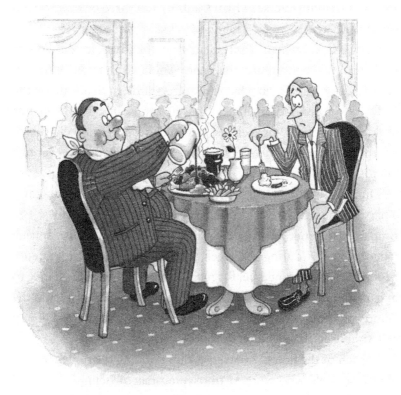

Feeding time

It got to the point where I was acutely embarrassed by the whole event and would feign tiredness, sickness or imaginary dates with the local hotties to avoid the inevitable questions and shifty looks that my dining habits were now attracting.

To make matters worse, my otherwise charming trips around the Welsh valleys were being increasingly spoiled by the eye-watering stomach spasms from the highway days. I was losing more weight and starting to look like the freshly sucked victim of the local vampire sect. It was at this stage that I discovered something I had never previously considered: Appetite is such a powerful mechanism that it cannot be overcome by willpower alone. Although I had never believed a word of this when trotted out by the fatties of the world, it is, in fact, true.

Although I could occasionally manage something of a decent breakfast on my better days, both lunch and dinner had become non-events for me. I would lecture myself as I drove between sales calls that I could and would eat a steak tonight. I had always liked steak, my stomach would be empty; surely I could put a piece of hot, juicy fillet steak in my mouth, chew it and swallow it, then repeat the exercise until the steak had gone? But I could not do it; I just could not do it.

I would be convinced I could achieve the feat right until the moment the food was placed in front of me, then both the sight and the smell would induce an overwhelming feeling of imminent vomiting. Although I might manage a piece or two on a good day, nothing on earth could persuade me to square the elbows and give it a good go. It also became apparent to me that another manifestation of this problem was that I didn't feel hungry – ever. No matter when or what I had last eaten, hunger pangs had gone from my life.

When you are feeling awful for a prolonged period, you can actually get used to it and subconsciously accept your circumstances as being relatively normal, which for you they are. This is compounded by the fact that it is natural to become inwardly focused and self-absorbed when feeling under the weather. These can combine and result in you losing any points of reference on what constitutes normality.

Tip #16 – Keep it Real

Keep your eyes open. If your dietary or bathroom habits are radically out of line with everyone around you, then something must be wrong. If you get up five times a night, every night, with the runs, that is not normal. If you never feel hungry and can never clear a plate, neither are those. Make sure your doctor registers just how far from the mainstream you have sunk.

What had happened was that my itinerant lifestyle had roused my Crohn's disease from its slumber to become far more aggressive than I had ever known it before. My symptoms were not caused by stress, but they were greatly worsened by the salesman's lifestyle that can be a test to the hardiest of constitutions, with irregular and fleeting lunches, lack of home comforts and being chucked out of dingy shops by idiotic retailers on a regular basis. Unfortunately, my mother was not given the chance to see for herself how fast I was declining as, due to the fact I was working away all week, I neither visited home nor allowed her to come down for the weekend, claiming that I would be too tired and too busy.

The one event that shocked me into action and finally forced me to reject the hoax diagnoses of stress, piles etc. was my return to the Cadbury's marketing department in May 1983. People there, for the most part, had not seen me for nine months and I was stunned to see how shocked most people were by my appearance. I had left a reasonably healthy-looking individual and returned looking like a dead man walking. You might wonder why this would be news to me, since I saw myself every day in the shaving mirror, but therein lies the problem.

Because you see yourself every day, you do not notice the gradual but inexorable shift in your appearance. Crohn's disease is insidious in that, apart from the odd blood-letting or pile-driver to the guts, it is not an illness of major events but of slow decline. While you might think you look a bit peaky on some mornings, you do not see the gradual disappearance of your body's precious stores of iron.

Tip #17 – Know Yourself

If you are worried that you might be getting worse, adopt the habit of regularly weighing yourself at the same time of day. Compare recent photos of yourself with ones from the recent past. This way you have factual evidence to present to your doctor that he will pay a lot more attention to than mumbled comments about not feeling as well as you did a while ago.

It took colleagues recoiling in horror to make me realize that I had been a passive patient for long enough. So I went to see the physician and would not leave his office until he had booked me an appointment with a gastroenterologist. This was the first time I realized that doctors, despite their airs of omnipotence and infallibility, will soon wilt if you manage the confrontation in the right way.

I am not advocating stand-up rows every time you visit your family doctor. They are well used to dealing with perpetually obnoxious people and rarely listen to a word being shouted at them.

However, used sparingly, a change in your attitude and showing resolute firmness can get the message through that this time they should reappraise the situation.

Tip #18: Draw a Line in the Sand

The first step is not to be overawed. The white coat, framed certificates on the wall, frosty and interfering receptionist ("Can I ask what it is you want to see him about?"), stethoscopic neckwear and large desk are a set of cleverly designed tools designed to keep us patients in a state of meek compliance. Once you ignore all that and start standing up for yourself, they are spent forces with nothing left in the tank. Even so, you have to stand your ground and make it clear that you will not be fobbed off with more of the same or "we'll see how it goes in the next couple of weeks." Ask for what you want: "I think I really need to see a specialist. This is not normal and is getting a lot worse."

A week later, I received through the post an appointment to see the gastroenterologist at the local hospital in four months' time. If I had kept this appointment, which I didn't, I probably wouldn't be sat here today typing this.

While going on the sales force had brought on a full-blown episode of the illness, my diagnosis and initial treatment owed everything to a random and long sequence of changes to my living arrangements back in Birmingham which culminated in my moving into a rented house, which I shared very happily with two wonderful people. Madeleine, who had joined Cadbury the same time as had I, worked in the rather austere-sounding group audit department where her role was to descend unannounced into other company departments and conduct financial audits to uncover the expense cheats.

The other housemate, Cheryl, had shared an apartment with another Cadbury friend and the huge stroke of luck was that she worked as a medical illustrator – a photographer in layman's terms – in Birmingham's Royal Free Hospital. On hearing that my hard-won appointment with the gastroenterologist at the local hospital was months away, Cheryl had approached a senior gastro-intestinal surgeon she worked with at the Royal Free and asked if he could help at all. He said that I should just come along to his weekly clinic the very next week.

Although I had not noticed until Cheryl stepped in, my battle with the as-yet-unidentified Crohn's had ceased to be a solitary one and had became one shared with supportive friends. Sharing a house with two very caring people was, in hindsight, a godsend at the time for which I am eternally grateful. I think now that I didn't divulge enough with them about how I was feeling, but both Madeleine and Cheryl could see that I was clearly not well, and each, in her own way, gave me the moral support that is absolutely essential in dealing with long-term illness.

Living with someone who has major eating problems cannot be easy. We took turns doing the cooking and I'm sure they must have found my efforts dull and somewhat repetitive given that I only had two recipes (lasagna and sweet & sour pork) that in any way stimulated my traumatized system. Equally, they never once complained about the fact that I would rarely, if ever, clear my plate when it was their respective turns.

Tip #19: Don't Reject or Bore your Friends

When ill with Crohn's, it can be very easy to either retreat into your shell or to become an illness bore. Either of these routes will deprive you of the full benefit that comes from having close, supportive friends. Involve friends in what is going on but don't pass the problem over to them with a "woe is me" attitude.

So I was delighted to hear that Cheryl had got me on the inside track. Not only was I jumping a very long queue, I would be going to see a better class of medical specialist as the Royal Free Hospital was one of Birmingham University's teaching hospitals, whereas I had been booked in at the local district hospital.

Tip #20: If There is a Queue, Jump It, but Look Before You Leap

These days, four-month waits are most unusual given the focus on reducing waiting lists, but even so, do not give up finding ways to jump the queue as just the act of seeking a quicker way in gives you the satisfaction of feeling like you are doing something positive. But do not sacrifice quality of care for speediness. Unless you are being ushered to the front of the queue by an insider, if you can get into another hospital tomorrow, ask yourself why they seemingly have no patients. Balance the length-of-wait goal with the need to get to see the very best people in the very best establishment. This is because not all doctors are equally skilled – someone qualified with the lowest pass-mark in the class, and probably at the fourth or fifth attempt – so these are the doctors you do not want to see. Do what I had failed to do: Conduct thorough research and insist that your family doctor send you where the doctors most competent in what ails you ply their trade. The British health service has a million employees, so you must know some- one who you can ask. Also, the fact that hospitals all have websites now is a great aid to doing your research.

But even with this breakthrough, there were still hurdles to deal with. On turning up to the weekly clinic at the Royal Free Hospital, I again fell foul of the spontaneity problem. Arriving without an official appointment, a letter from my physician or a bulging folder of notes meant that I sat there for three hours being ignored by everyone until they were shutting up shop and I was the last person there. Some kindly soul eventually enquired what I thought I was doing, and, although they claimed to know nothing of my invitation, did a full consultation. The outcome of a fresh and highly qualified pair of ears hearing my tale of woe was the booking of the barium meal that was to eventually lead to my diagnosis.

So, if I had not had the immense good fortune to be sharing a house with Cheryl, I would have waited another four months only to see probably the least competent gastro-intestinal specialist in the whole of Birmingham. I am not sure how I could have survived another four months of my symptoms by that point. It was due to Cheryl's initiative in getting me into the Birmingham Royal Free, albeit by the back door, that led directly to my diagnosis and initial encounter with Dr Ray described in Chapter 1. To bring the story bang up-to-date: Dr. Ray ended that meeting by telling me that I needed immediate surgery. At last things were moving.

The News Sinks In

"I told you I was ill"
– Tombstone

AS I LEFT Doctor Ray's office following our initial impromptu meeting, I felt as though I was walking on air. The confirmation of a firm diagnosis above all else gave me a supreme sense of vindication. I had not been making it up, nor had I been stressed, nor had I been unable to look after myself – I had a genuine medical condition. The fact that it had taken medical science seven years to recognize it did not bother me at that moment; I was just delighted not to be to blame. It was like hearing the jury foreman say, "Not guilty" despite there having been a host of prosecution witnesses dramatically point to me when asked to identify the culprit.

My first action was to find the pay phone in the main hospital reception area and call my mother with the news.

"How did it go?"

"Great news Mom, they have diagnosed me for definite."

"Really? With what....?"

"Crohn's disease!!!!!! Isn't that marvelous????????"

"......................"

"Mom? Mom? You still there?"

My mother, being a medical professional of many years' standing, was not quite as ecstatic as was I at the news because she knew what lay ahead, whereas I, in my innocence, assumed that the heavy lifting was over and that I faced a symptom-free future by having the accumulated wisdom of the medical world at my disposal. Her reserve would begin to be justified almost immediately.

Not ten minutes previously, Dr. Ray's parting shot had been to confirm that the only treatment for the strictures in my small bowel was surgery and that "they would be in touch." Communicating this to my mother had generated another prolonged silence as, once again, she had more info than did I on what such surgery would entail. By now, as you can imagine, my initial euphoria had begun to wane somewhat. The feeling of having been declared "Not guilty" had been replaced by the grim realization that I was about to be rearrested on the steps of the courthouse.

Walking out of the Royal Free Hospital, as I pondered the not-so-subliminal message from my mother that my problems might not quite be over, my mind wandered to what would prove to be the most difficult part of succeeding at being ill: How do you combine an ongoing illness with the need to build a career or, at the very least, remain in paid employment? What would this mean back in the workplace?

A few weeks previously, I had returned to Cadbury's head office from my sales force odyssey and begun a new job as brand manager. This was a promotion from the job I had left nine months earlier and, thus far, a complete vindication of my decision to go and carry the sales bag. But what should I tell my new boss when I returned to the office the next day? "I'm going to be off work for I don't know how long, commencing I don't know when" would not be too welcome since I had only just arrived back, and equally not much use to him in planning around my absence. I clearly needed more information in preparation for this encounter.

This being in the pre-internet era, some leg-work was in order. A slight detour on my walk from the Royal Free Hospital took me to the Birmingham Central Library. Here, after some prolonged navigation into its deeper recesses, I found the medical section and located what seemed like a good primer on Inflammatory Bowel disease, a grouping which includes Crohn's disease, and settled down for a couple of hours to do a bit of homework.

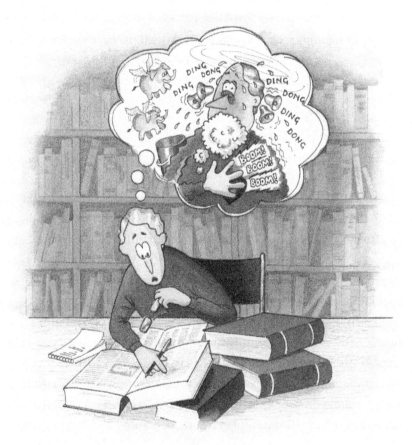

A textbook case

Tip #21: Learn About Crohn's

Medical textbooks and websites are not designed for the faint-hearted, and you should think hard before you open one as they seem to glory in the gory, judging by the space devoted to obscure side effects, gut-churning possible complications and seemingly endless mortality statistics. It can come as quite a shock to see so many daunting life possibilities laid out in front of you. However, because you will face choices over courses of treatments, the more clued up you are the better able you will be to exercise control over your destiny. It's up to you as to how much of the gory details you can take, but my recommendation is to push yourself to your limits. Best not to look at the pictures though; they are never helpful.

Despite blanching at some of the more worrisome complications of Crohn's disease, I found my research visit helpful. The medical profession, as a rule, works on the principle that you are better off knowing as little as possible because you will only worry. But ignorance is not a sound basis for successfully managing an illness such as Crohn's.

Even if they are believers in medical perestroika, you don't get much of it from five-minute consultations with doctors who are already three hours behind on their clinic list. Should you be fortunate enough to have your doctor's attention for more than a millisecond, you usually learn nothing as I have found their default communication mode to patients is to assume you are an idiot. Doctors do not hesitate to explain things in terms that would shame a Grade 1 teacher. To illustrate the point by jumping ahead slightly, immediately prior to my first surgery, the most detailed description I was given as to what would take place was, "We'll have a good root around, and if we see something we don't like the look of, we'll snip it out."

Your doctor assumes you are an idiot because, as anyone who works with the general public will confirm, there are a lot of idiots out there. My cousin, who works as a bank clerk, tells me that at least 90% of her customers are, to varying degrees, loopy. So it is understandable if your doctor's default assumption is that you are also probably a bit loopy and hence incapable of understanding complex medical conditions.

Tip #22: Convince Your Doctor You Are Not an Idiot

Establish early on in your doctorial relationship that you are not one of the clueless herd. By the questions you ask, showcase your understanding of your condition. They won't like it at first, but will gradually warm to the idea that you are capable of engaging in an intelligent conversation about your illness and the treatment options.

After the initial queasiness brought on by the gastroenterology textbooks had passed, I did learn enough in the library to be able to go back to work the next day with a slightly more coherent battle plan on how to manage the company's expectations on what would be happening. Although I wasn't able to give a date from which I would be absent, I had discovered that a small bowel operation was a big deal, this being in the days before the allegedly miracle technique of laparoscopy. Having your abdominal cavity opened up; your twenty-odd feet of small bowel manhandled from one end to the other and various bits chopped out was not a quick procedure: two to four hours was the guideline. That length of time under a general anesthetic knocks you back, adding weeks to your recovery time. So it was looking like I would be away for three to four months.

While this was not the best news my new boss would receive the next day, it at least would give a steer on what would be required to cope with such an absence. So prolonged was going to be my absence that the work clearly could not be allowed to pile up for my return, nor could it reasonably be doled out to my colleagues to cover. If it was for three or four weeks, then maybe they would muddle through, but three or four months meant that I had to come to terms with the fact that someone else would be doing my job and it may not be there for me when I returned.

The meeting went well. It was made clear to me that all that mattered was my health and that they would cope. We agreed that the job would have to be done full-time by someone else and that, closer to my return date, we would have to discuss other possible vacancies, not unlike the process that had take place to facilitate my transfer back from the sales force.

I have since met many fellow sufferers who ended up losing their jobs because of the amount of time they were taking off, and many had found it very difficult to get back into the workforce. I was lucky that I was working in a large enough organization where I was a very small cog in a very large wheel so my absence would not sink the ship.

Tip #23: Safety in Numbers

If your absences could cripple your employer, it is unreasonable of you to expect them to bear such a burden. Get yourself into as large an employer as possible. Even if you have to compromise your ideal job to be with an employer where your absences can more easily be borne, it is a compromise worth making.

Even so, it was a very big frustration that I was unable to tell my employer when this prolonged absence would commence. I understand that, especially these days, scheduling of surgery is a day-to-day process as they strive for 100% bed occupancy rates, but if I could change one thing about the health profession, it would be to get them to realize that you have a life and a career too, and that you don't have as much flexibility as they seem to imagine.

This is an annoyance that bedevils you throughout every aspect of living with Crohn's disease. I have spent countless hours waiting for what I was led to believe were scheduled appointments. Doctors' secretaries are serial over-bookers who put even the shoddiest airlines to shame. I have had it explained to me that doctors' time is so precious and patients are so unreliable they cannot take the slightest risk that the doctor is temporarily unemployed, even for a minute. Doctors save lives you know! Or so I am told.

However, I can report that, in the thousands of hours I have spent sitting awaiting long-overdue appointments, I have never seen a life saved, a Code Blue resuscitation, a Heimlich maneuver or even a Band-Aid applied to a cut finger, so I have yet to work out just why there seems to be such a vast disparity between the value of my time and that of the doctor's. And it's not just bowel doctors who place such a high value on their time. I understand why I might not be seen instantly in the emergency department, but at the dermatologist's? "URGENT MOLE IN ROOM THREE!", or the foot clinic? "LET ME THROUGH, I'M A PODIATRIST!!!"

As it turned out, my wait to hear the date of my operation would be ended not by a sudden outburst of forward planning in the Royal Free Hospital bed management department but by the onset of an even more crippling side effect of the illness. Not that I knew that's what it was when I awoke in the middle of the night with an excruciating pain in my nether regions. This was a pain that dwarfed all that had gone before; I was unable to move or even, it seemed for a while, breathe.

My mind raced with options as to what I should do. I soon decided that the extra pain involved in beginning breathing again was a cross I should consider bearing as the room began to go fuzzy at the edges. As my head cleared, my best plan seemed to be to bang on the wall behind my bed which separated my room from Madeleine's. But I quickly decided this might well strain our friendship beyond bounds. Firstly, my clock told me it was 3am, so being awoken by mysterious banging on her wall might not be too well received.

But what would I ask her to do even if I did rouse her? The pain was coming from much further down than the usual obstruction pain; in fact it was centered right between my legs, in the perianal area to be clinically precise, between Number Onesy and Number Twosy. While Madeleine was, and is, a very good friend, I'm not sure how she would have reacted to "Take a close look down there and see what is so painful. You might have to feel for something!" So I reverted to Plan B, which was to wait it out until morning and hope that the pain would lessen sufficiently for me to be able to get out of bed.

Svelte mothers who have had to deliver gargantuan babies will appreciate the feeling of pain that seems will last a lifetime while being unbearable for another five minutes. The four hours until getting up time seemed like forever. How do you bear the unbearable? I have no good advice to offer; you just bear it because there is no alternative, no escape.

I could find no alternative position that in any way eased the pain, even a fraction. My mental happy places soon became barren deserts. Just when I thought I had been consigned to the worst dungeon of Hell for all eternity, I heard stirring in the house; Madeleine and Cheryl were getting up.

The only upside of my circumstances was that tentative movements made me realize that, the pain being so bad, movement didn't actually make it any worse: I think my pain receptors were working on maximum loading. So I crawled out of bed and all but slid down the stairs on my side which came as something of a surprise to my housemates as they chatted over their muesli. Since they both knew I had not gone on a complete bender the night before, I avoided the accusation of still being drunk, even though I must have sounded and looked like it. As soon as the family doctor's surgery opened, I was on the phone demanding a home visit, a wish that was mercifully granted.

The girls had sensibly suggested leaving the door unlocked and giving the doctor instructions to let himself in, which he did soon after his morning clinic had finished. If he was surprised to find me lying on my stomach with my legs flipped up in the air, he didn't show it; I'm sure they get to see some worse sights. Due to my relative helplessness, he did the honors in debagging me of my pajamas and then whipped out his pen/flashlight prior to parting my cheeks like the Red Sea. A preliminary jab with his index finger evoked an eardrum-splitting howl.

"Tender, is it?" As you may have gathered by now, my GP was a man of few words. In response he heard sobs muffled by cushion-biting strong enough to shear steel girders.

"I'll take that as a 'yes' then."

The diagnosis came very quickly in comparison to the seven years taken to solve the Crohn's puzzle: He immediately declared it to be an abscess buried deep in the perianal tissue and informed me that this was a relatively uncommon symptom of Crohn's disease.

He then correctly divined my muffled groaning to be a request of information on treatment options, ideally rapid ones.

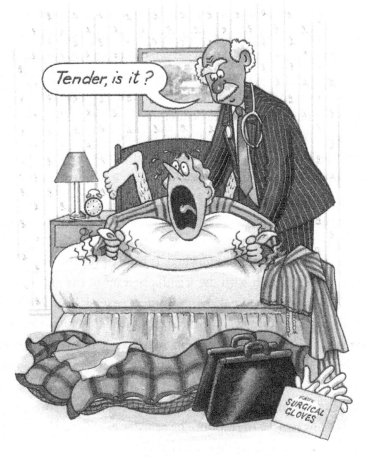

Tender in the night

"It needs draining, so, given you are seeing Dr. Ray at the Royal Free for your Crohn's, you should give him a call."

This was not what I wanted to hear – couldn't it be fixed now? Apparently not. His heart wasn't made completely of stone though;

he did leave a bottle of weapons-grade painkillers to get me through the ordeal.

After the family doctor had skedaddled, I called Dr. Ray's secretary and managed to give her the gist of the situation, and was promised that she would update him with this latest development as soon as possible. This, you might think, would automatically result in my being bumped up the waiting list and there be a summons that day, or, at worst, the next, to come on into Ward 8 for corrective action. Well, that's what I thought, but more fool me. Days passed with me still crippled by this increasingly large abscess, by now the size of a grade A goose egg, with no news from Ward 8 and the family doctor having literally and figuratively washed his hands of me. It only gradually dawned on me that each must have thought the other was going to sort it out.

I have found that doctors seem to worry greatly about initiating territorial disputes with other doctors. So it is not uncommon for their default action to be to leave the problem to the other guy to sort out. When you get your appointment with your specialist, you may well be told, "I don't know why he didn't send you to xxxx; you need to make an appointment there." You can spend years not being treated for something if there is confusion as to whether or not it is related to your illness.

Tip #24: Beware of Demarcation Issues

Do not automatically accept the buck being passed. Ask specifically if this particular problem will definitely be addressed by the specialist. When you call the specialist's office, do not just book an appointment but ask if that is the correct course of action to get the particular issue resolved.

This lack of a sense of urgency in Ward 8 did not go down well with my mother, who had driven down to Birmingham that day to be closer to the action. She could not hide her horror at seeing the abscess for herself, declaring it to be clearly in need of urgent treatment. She then took it upon herself to clear the logjam by ringing the Ward 8 nurse and forcefully impressing on her the exact status of this pulsating mass. Phone calls from my mother are not easily ignored, so the very next day I received a terse letter from the hospital telling me to present myself at the admissions department the day after.

Medics and their protective screen of secretaries are much more likely to take a call from someone within their own profession – they are a bit masonic that way. There's no point you doing it yourself as you have more chance of a miracle cure than you do of getting past the Obersturmbahnfuhrer in the outer office; patients do not get a vote in the running of hospitals. Given that the British National Health Service has over 1.3 million employees, one is almost certain to know someone on the inside. You can spot them if you know the signs to look out for. Anyone who calls stitches sutures or refers to your collarbone as your clavicle is inadvertently giving himself away. If you hear him refer to the far end of something as distal (Example: "I'll meet you in the distal carriage on the train"), then you have struck gold.

Tip #25: Get an Insider on Your Team

If you know anyone at all who is on the inside, then sign them up to your cause and rope them in to conduct negotiations with the medics. And if you are truly blessed in knowing more than one such person, don't sign up the shrinking violet of the two; you are going to need all the firepower you can get.

So it seemed my salvation from the crippling rear-end pain was at hand. That I would also be undergoing a massive and complex surgical procedure was a mere afterthought in comparison. The next day I packed my bag with what I thought were the essential components of a hospital survival kit: plenty to read; plenty to listen to; plenty to suck and the most voluminous and modest flannel pajamas I possessed – this was no time for silk boxers and more erection-phobia. If the taxi driver was surprised by the inflatable rubber ring I brought along to ease the trip, he didn't show it. So off I chugged to the next phase of my medical journey and a long-overdue encounter with the scalpel.

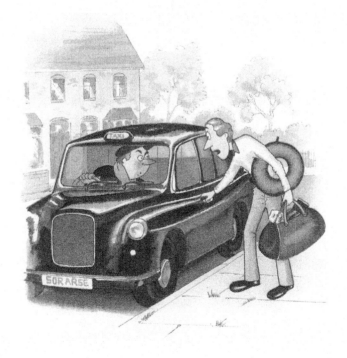

"...and go very slowly over the speed bumps!"

Waiting Patiently

"It seems a very strange principle to enunciate as the very first requirement in a hospital that it should do the sick no harm."

– Florence Nightingale, Nurse (1820 – 1910)

AFTER SUCCESSFULLY NAVIGATING the Royal Free's check-in process perched on the edge of the seat using the outer half of one buttock, I hobbled up to Ward 8 still in a positive frame of mind. The abscess and the digestive pains had me in such despair that I would have signed up for literally anything if it meant being able to sit down and enjoy food again. The only thing on my mind was wondering what the facilities would be like as it was clear I would be living here for more than a few days. During my previous visit, I had not got past Dr. Ray's office, so I had no idea what my actual accommodation would look like, although I think I had a default assumption that it would look like the set from a 1950s movie where nurses wearing starched aprons policed long wards full of cheery fellow medical travelers.

As I approached the nurses' room beyond Dr Ray's office, it was apparent that the ward, which was situated at one end of the building, was T-shape in layout with the sleeping quarters being split into two on either side of nursing mission control. I was treated to a guided tour by the ward sister – Sister Grey – of the right-hand leg of the ward which was the men's domain. The ladies were effectively off-limits through some double doors on the left, their modesty preserved from any prying male eyes by frosted glass windows.

As I entered the men's side, I did indeed see what looked just like the archetypal ward I had in mind, which is known in the trade as a Nightingale Ward, named after but not invented by Florence herself. Sister Grey clearly ran a tight ship as nurses visibly quickened their pace as we came in. There were five beds on each side of the ward, which was a very bright room illuminated by tall windows between each bed. The walls were that peculiar shade of institutional pale green, of which there must have been at least a dozen coats applied over time. The manufacturer must have delivered it by the tanker-full as that had been the only color visible throughout my journey from the hospital entrance.

At the far end was situated a bathroom; two toilets and the "sluice room" where bedpans and sick bowls were washed out. There was also what appeared to be a room with a door glazed from waist height to ceiling with frosted glass, through which I could vaguely see some seated figures. As Sister opened the door into this mysterious lair, it was immediately apparent that the glass was in fact perfectly clear, the room being enveloped in a Dickensian pea-souper of cigarette smoke coming from the five inhabitants who were all vigorously puffing away as though they were majority shareholders in R. J. Reynolds. Apparently this was the TV room, though I had to take Sister Grey's word that the shadowy flickering in the far corner of the room was in fact a normally functioning television.

This hospital equivalent of the school stairway accounted for the fact that the ward had seemed almost deserted of patients. There were only three beds actually occupied which meant that, including the smokers' union, I had a choice of two spare beds that could be my new home, this being years before the arrival of hospital administrators and their target 135% bed occupancy rates. I plumped for one nearer to the entrance, my reasoning being that I should be quite safe from the fog that drifted from the TV room every time someone came up for air. This being a men's ward, my welcome from my fellow inmates consisted of either a brief nod or, from the chatty types, a "Hi".

Tip #26: Choose Your Friends Carefully

In the hospital setting, there is no escape once you have established contact. Striking up a conversation before you have had a chance to evaluate the personality type can be an invitation to being endlessly bored. If you enjoy talking to absolutely anyone then I would thoroughly recommend rushing to make friends with one's fellow inmates as a course of action. If, however, you are like me and value stimulating conversation as opposed to being talked at, then it is the worst thing you can do.

Sister Grey, a middle-aged lady with a kindly face that exuded cool professionalism, suggested I get unpacked and changed into my pajamas, pulling the curtain around as she did so. She then informed me that, as ward rounds had already finished, it could be quite a while before one of the junior members of the surgical "firm" who would be slicing me open would be round to interrogate me.

Once I was into my overly modest night attire, I sat on the bed and surveyed my domain. A small bedside table, an emergency button and an ancient set of earphones coated with several years' worth of what I presumed to be human earwax seemed to be the only items of potential usability, so I jammed my clothes into the cupboard part of the table, laid out and wired up my entertainment centre, which consisted of a newly purchased personal stereo and a pile of cassette tapes, drew back the curtain, then sat on the bed to await events. Cleaning the earphones would not be a quick job, so would have to wait. Thirty minutes later, I had already divined the main feature of being a hospital in-patient: Nothing happens for exceptionally long periods of time.

Tip #27: Make the Fun Last as Long as Possible

Never rush anything; in fact, stretch out every activity such as reading or crosswords as long as you can. In between activities, take a keen interest in the workings of the ward by finding a seat in one of the public areas.

I am completely anti being in the private room where, in my experience, the inmate spends the whole of his stay feeling desperately sorry for himself. In a shared ward, even a two-bedded one, not only is there more going on but there is a 50% chance one of your fellow inmates will be far worse off than you, so you feel lucky to not be in their shoes, which is good for your morale. If he is not as ill as you, he will soon be evicted and replaced by someone who is.

Tip #28: Avoid Solitary Confinement

If you are going to be in for anything longer than one night, don't book a private room. Paying more money to feel more miserable is not a good investment. Solitary is a punishment in prison for a reason.

As the smokers' union filtered back into what must have seemed to them a world of terrifying clarity and brightness, the ward soon busied with a gaggle of nurses completing various tasks. At first glance, there appeared to be three ranks in the nursing pecking order: Sister Grey, who wore a royal blue uniform; a couple of staff (i.e. qualified) nurses dressed in white uniforms, who always seemed to stride purposefully towards whatever task was next, and several, younger-looking nurses dressed in pale blue uniforms, who I correctly divined to be students. They were the chatty ones, both between themselves and with the patients, and most came over to my bed to introduce themselves and ask if I was settling in. On quizzing a particularly chirpy one, I discovered there was a further ranking system within the students, denoted by the number of small blue bands on the upper part of their white caps: one band for a first-year student, two for second-year and three for third and final year. It seems everyone needs someone to look down upon.

Once I had scoped the ward staffing arrangements, I turned my attentions to what had become the most pressing matter on my mind: cleaning the earphones of their caked-on layers of wax. This preoccupied me for a good hour, and consumed my entire stock of facial tissues, plus gave me a life-long antipathy to other people's ear wax. Why the previous occupants had accepted the waxy status quo, I have no idea. Was it just me? Do others see ear wax as being like recently vacated warm seats: clearly of human origin but lacking any euugghh factor? Or perhaps the layers of wax formed an immediate bond with the wearer's own supply, ensuring that the earphones would not fall out should the wearer nod off, a problem I never managed to solve to my full satisfaction with my personal stereo.

Nearing the end of the final ear-piece buffing and polishing, I was interrupted by the arrival of a doctor, who quite self-importantly announced herself as the "junior houseman". Luckily, I had been briefed a couple of days earlier by my mother as to what the various ranks of doctors actually did, so I remained uncowed. The junior houseman was the lowest of the low - a spear-carrying member of the chorus line – fresh out of medical school and keen to save humanity, but their spirit already crushed by being trusted with only the most menial of tasks while having to work 160-hour weeks. Her responsibility on this occasion, it transpired, was to take my history; more senior doctors finding it beneath them to talk to new patients.

As I was giving her chapter and verse on the events of the previous seven years, she expressed surprise that I was sounding so upbeat. Not that I wasn't feeling physically dreadful – I was – but there was no doubt that my spirits seemed to be several levels higher than she had been expecting. Apparently, my mother, while giving Sister Grey a severe telephone-bashing to get me admitted, had painted a bleak picture as to my current state, so much so that the junior houseman seemed to have been expecting little more than a walking corpse. This apparently inconsequential fact illuminates a couple of key insights for the successful patient-to-be.

Firstly, once you are in hospital, you have hundreds of billions of dollars-worth of people, experience and equipment working on your behalf. The hard bit, though, is getting in. When you are in dire straits, it is not the time to be bashful. You must drop your reserve and adopt the law of the jungle. Once you are in, you will most likely not be sent away until you have been treated in some way. Even though I was clearly in better shape than the doctor had been expecting, no one was going to send me home again until they had taken the chance to open me up.

Tip #29: Hospitals are Full of Doctors, Nurses and Technology That Can Help You

Don't turn down the option, if offered, of being admitted to hospital. Yes, it is not pleasant, but you are much more likely to have your condition improved. But take steps to protect yourself from getting hospital infections. Don't be afraid to tell people to wash their hands before they come near you.

Secondly, far from feeling depressed at the prospect of having to undergo major surgery, I was very positive about it, as I have been for all subsequent surgeries. This is because surgery is usually the solution rather than the problem. You only need surgery when you are self-evidently quite ill and most likely feeling pretty rotten. In that situation, the only way is up. In my case I was seeing surgery as being my imminent salvation from the daily grind of gripping pain and awful appetite.

Tip #30: See Surgery as a Solution, Not a Problem

By all means worry beforehand about how to stay out of the hands of the surgeons if you can endure your symptoms, but once you have to undergo the knife, think positively. Surgical patients who approach the ordeal with a positive mindset have fewer complications and recover faster than those who are completely depressed by the prospect, so to some extent your fate is within your own hands.

As I neared the end of relating to the junior assistant trainee surgeon my Homeric health saga, I brought up the issue of the still extremely painful abscess in my nethers. This prompted an immediate drawing of the curtains and forcible insertion of a gigantic red-hot poker into my anus, or at least that's what I assumed had happened, though it turned out that only the gentlest of prods had brought about my latest journey into the land that pain relief forgot. However, it clearly brightened up the junior houseman's day. Here was something new she could relay back to her masters, giving her the opportunity to demonstrate her many doctorly qualities in recommending a suitable course of action. So off she trotted for reinforcements.

Fifteen minutes later I had quite an audience, all keenly interested in my rear end; I could have sold tickets. After they had been huddled for a while, the beaming junior houseman extricated herself to deliver the prognosis: I couldn't have the operation while this pulsating mass of pus was so near the critical area, as post-operative infection would be virtually guaranteed. The consensus was that it would have to be drained the next day.

While I was upbeat about major abdominal surgery, the prospect of rear-end abscess-draining did not sound so good. Would I be awake? What if I sneezed at the wrong moment with a razor-sharp scalpel less than an inch away from my heat-seeking love missile? What if the scalpel-wielder sneezed at the critical moment? These thoughts brought on an involuntary cheek-clenching which only racked up the rear-end painometer to new levels.

As it turned out, I was to be spared the draining procedure. I escaped because, that evening, I eagerly took up the offer of a sleeping tablet from the oncoming night nursing staff. It had become clear quite early in the evening that sharing a room with eight other men, all of whom were at least forty years older than me, was not going to be a restful nocturnal experience. Everyone was already coughing, scratching, farting or snoring, some accomplishing all four simultaneously. This is without doubt the biggest downside of being in a shared ward, but is far outweighed by the benefits of the increased daytime mental stimulation.

Tip #31: Always Take the Sleeping Tablets

Never, ever, turn down the offer of a sleeping tablet in hospital. While you may be feeling quite sleepy and the ward is as quiet as the grave, neither will be the case for eight hours. At three in the morning, listening to your neighbors' orifices compete with each other to set new loudness records, you would happily kill just to get ten minutes' sleep. This is the most common reason for requesting a private room, but while those in shared wards can take a sleeping tablet at night, those in their isolation cells can't take an anti-boredom and misery tablet during the day.

No doubt, long experience had taught the staff that industrial-strength sleeping tablets were required to get patients through the night, with the not inconsequential benefit to themselves that a sleeping ward is one that requires less work. So strong were the tablets that I must have adopted a sleeping position that put undue pressure on the abscess without awakening myself. The pressure burst the abscess, forcing an opening in my skin and spraying my lower half and the bed sheets with pus.

I don't actually remember this happening. I only became aware of it as I groggily came to in the morning in the same way that Jack Woltz, the movie producer in The Godfather who wouldn't give Johnny Fontane the part, moved from being perplexed to worried to downright terrified as he discovered he was covered in blood seeping from the horse's head in his bed. I went on a similar emotional rollercoaster as it became apparent that I had seemingly been attacked by the Ghostbusters during the night. I had no idea why my legs were soaked in a sticky mess. But instead of yelling the place down as well I might, I merely pressed the emergency button and awaited the arrival of the cavalry. I didn't want my fellow ward residents to mark me down as the hysterical type.

Perhaps my emergency should be called a Code Green as I had never seen so much green goo in my life; even the nursing staff that came to investigate my alarm call were visibly impressed. I can't imagine how I would have reacted if this had happened while I was still at home, or in the taxi going to the hospital. The nurses cleaned me up and then went in for a closer examination like volcanologists investigating Mount Etna's latest eruption. Where there had been a large, very angry-looking lump, it was now back to normal apart from there being a little round hole, as though made by a hole punch, through which the green magma had erupted.

The staff nurse pronounced that, with a dressing on, it'd be right as rain in a couple of days when I would be cleared for surgery. The junior houseman was summoned to confirm the prognosis, although I could barely tell what she was mumbling as apparently she hadn't been to sleep since our discussion the previous day. These were the good old days of junior doctors working days on end without a break.

She looked even worse when I saw her again an hour or so later, as this time she was accompanied by the rest of the surgical firm, together with a few students. The firm consisted of herself at the foot of the totem pole right up to the head man, via the senior houseman, junior registrar, senior registrar, ending up with the consultant surgeon himself. He was straight from Central Casting: the dashing king of the scalpel-wielders; supremely self-confident and clearly master of all he surveyed. A clean-cut, energetic man who I would have put at a young-looking early 60s, he approached my bed while regaling his team with an anecdote about having been summonsed the previous evening from a dinner to remove a stomach ulcer the size of a quail's egg. I imagined he had conducted the operation while still wearing his white tie and tails, then managed to get back in time for the cheese and port. He definitely had the look of someone who fearlessly sliced people open fully confident he could put the right bits back together again.

The scene played out with the extremely nervous and exhausted junior houseman giving a summary of my case, while constantly being interrupted by the God, as he lectured the assembled throng on some hitherto unrealized aspect of surgery for Crohn's disease. He threw in a few witticisms which, although generating widespread chortles and murmurs of appreciation from the white-coat brigade, seemed less than funny to me, mainly because they appeared to be delivered mostly in Latin. Jokes about the distal jejunum would not play well at Caesar's Palace, but they seemed to go down a storm around my bed. I decided to hold my tongue as I was learning nothing from his comedic routine and the patient doesn't get a speaking part at these events anyway.

When you have a crowd of doctors around your bed, you have to recognize that this is their show and not yours. The top dog needs to demonstrate his profound knowledge to his minions; the junior doctors need to demonstrate their proficiency on the basics of your case, and the medical students need to concentrate fiercely, not just to learn from the Master, but to memorize the next steps he will at some stage pronounce. You, on the other hand, might as well be a tailor's dummy. I have invariably found it counter-productive to interrupt the proceedings while they are in full flow. The initial response to your, "Excuse me, but I was just wondering…" is exactly as though you had done a very loud fart at the dinner table. There is a silent pause while all eyes seek you out, then, after you have been glared at by all, their conversation resumes as though your dreadful faux pas had never happened.

Tip #32: Pay Attention, But Don't Interrupt.

But your time should not be wasted. It is wise to pay close attention to what is being said as you will have the opportunity to quiz the trainees once the show has finished to explain further what exactly lies immediately ahead for you.

After finishing with my case, he strode over to the next bed with his acolytes in tow like a small flotilla of ducklings, leaving the second banana, the senior registrar, to give me the English translation which I could quiz him upon.

Because my Crohn's had been diagnosed largely by chance, and I was now occupying a bed for at least a couple of days before the knife could be wielded, they were going to take the opportunity to do a more thorough examination of my digestive tract to search for any other manifestations of the disease. Crohn's disease, he said, could affect not just the small bowel (the twenty-two feet of small intestine) but also the large bowel (the subsequent portion prior to the rectum), so they wanted to check it out. Apparently, perianal abscesses were associated with the disease having spread to that area. Having delivered that piece of good news with a suitably deadpan demeanor, he toddled off to join the doctoral scrum now around the bed to my right.

Another member of the throng that had been round my bed, Sister Grey, had also hung back and now followed up with the nitty-gritty. I could not have anything to eat or drink, aside from water, for the next twenty-four hours, which immediately set me sobbing inside. I knew from bitter experience that this was a sure sign of another encounter with the barium milkshakes.

"Not quite," said Sister Grey, "There will be barium, but it'll be going in the other end as an enema."

"Well that's a relief," said I. She smiled and patted my arm, but in her eyes I could see a look of deep sorrow that filled me with a nameless dread.

The day passed completely uneventfully until later in the afternoon when the senior registrar returned saying that he had a favor to ask of me. Since I had spent much of the intervening period glumly considering what might be involved in undergoing a barium enema, I wasn't sure that I should be signing up for any more of his suggestions, but I let him make his case. It transpired that it was exam time for medical students in their final year (the Royal Free was one of the teaching hospitals for Birmingham University's medical school), and a key part of the test was for students to have twenty minutes to examine an anonymous patient, after which they were to pronounce diagnosis. I have to admit this piqued my interest and it would fill up an hour or two.

To avoid giving the students the unmissable clue of examining me in the Inflammatory Bowel disease specialist ward that was Ward 8, I was escorted up a floor and given a bed in a general ward, where I awaited the first nervous student. The process was to be repeated four times and each followed a similar path. The student would give me a thorough once-over and then quiz me based on the general area in which they thought my health problem lay, all the while being subjected to eye-rolling, sighing and the occasional, "Good God, man!" from the examiner.

Needless to say, not one of the students even got as far as identifying the digestive tract as being the source of my problems, let alone nailing Crohn's disease. At twenty-minute intervals I was variously pronounced with unshakeable confidence as suffering from heart disease, liver failure, cancer, kidney stones and something I'm sure I heard as Ron Atkinson's disease, although why the then Manchester United manager would have a disease named after him I had no idea. After each "diagnosis", the examiner would demolish their diagnostic technique and identify the various pointers to Crohn's disease in a tone of voice that indicated he thought a child of five playing Doctors and Nurses would have spotted it in three minutes tops. Feeling sorry for their broken spirits, I would mutter to them as they finished up that it had taken seven years for their betters to reach a correct diagnosis of me, so they should not be too disheartened.

But the exercise, while meeting the objective of keeping me distracted for a couple of hours, did have a downside. After I was deposited back in Ward 8, I began to worry. What if these medical novices had spotted something that had been missed by the many doctors I had seen during the last seven years? If the experts could miss a seemingly obvious case of Crohn's for all that time, what else might they have missed? What if I really did have heart disease, liver disease, cancer, kidney stones or Big Ron's disease and the Ward 8 specialists were too fixated on having identified Crohn's to see the wood for the trees? A bit like the police pursuing their usual suspects while ignoring the written, signed confession from the husband pinned to the wife's body. Tunnel vision happens all the time.

This bout of justifiable hypochondria would be swept away the next day when the barium enema took my mind away from theoretical worries and back to more practical issues such as legalized medical torture. If you want to stop worrying about having to undergo a barium meal, have a barium enema first – it's ten times worse, even though you don't have to drink the sludge.

The process begins by completely stripping away any remaining shreds of your dignity. As usual, you are vulnerably naked beneath the oversize gown with the added feature that you are face down with your butt sticking in the air. But it's not all bad news: at least you don't have to watch the approach of the implement that will soon be inserted within, like some poor terrified wretch watching Vincent Price approach with the thumbscrews. The tube itself can't be too wide a bore as it goes in without excessive eye-watering, and then the initial flow of the liquid barium is something you hardly perceive at all. All would be well if this was the extent of the procedure, but for the radiographer to get good pictures on the X-ray machine, she needs to dilate your large bowel to several times life size, a feat she accomplishes with the use of compressed air.

Just as I was wondering what the hissing noise was, I found out the hard way as enough air was pumped into me to inflate the tires of a Mack 16-wheeler.

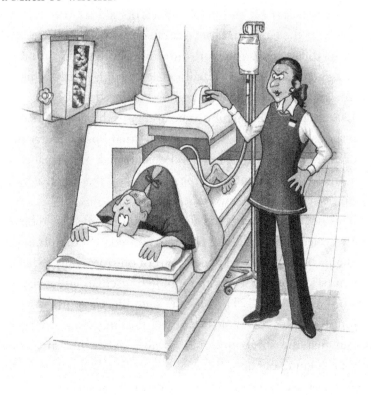

The perils of hyper-inflation

When you think you will either explode or faint from the intense discomfort, your system submits and goes into reverse, allowing the air to pass further upstream. This natural safety valve lessens the pain – although you still feel as bloated as the Goodyear blimp – but then your relief that the worst may be over is swept away as you get another top-up from the 30psi line. This is repeated time after time, all the while being exhorted by the staff not to let pass any of the by now barium equivalent of a very well shaken bottle of Diet Coke seeded with three packets of Mentos. So you clench your cheeks as though attempting to crack walnuts and try not to imagine the ignominy of pebble-dashing the entire room.

The procedure seems to last forever, but it does of course finally pass, as does the largest fart of your life once you are ushered to the adjoining toilet where you hang onto the seat to avoid shooting up to the ceiling like a badly tied balloon at a birthday party. This really was the worst medical procedure I had endured to date.

Later that day, the suction-tube holder of the surgical team, the junior houseman, returned with the news that I had undergone this torture for nothing: my large bowel was normal, or normal enough not to need the sharp edge of the scalpel, and that my real surgery was to be scheduled for two days hence.

This final delay was so the abscess ejection hole would be sufficiently healed and my digestive system cleared. After returning from the enema, I had managed to eat a part of one meal only to have the staff nurse follow up from the junior houseman and once again hang on my bed the "Nil by Mouth" sign. I faced another two days without food plus the explosive bowel-flushing. I was now getting so thin that the surgeon would be able to see my small bowel without opening me up.

But, at least we could finally get down to business.

The First Cut Is The Deepest

"Minor surgery is surgery someone else is having"
   — **J. Carl Cook**

I AWOKE ON what was a beautiful June morning with the sun
streaming into the ward, illuminating the crocodile of farting old
men hobbling down towards the two toilets. I had enjoyed another
good night's sleep thanks to the usual dose of sleeping tablets, so
my worrying about undergoing surgery for the first time had not
been as prolonged as it might have been. I was up for it. Bring on
the pain!

The only real question on my mind was regarding my position
on the surgery batting order. This was soon answered by the
surgical team's dogsbody, who came round soon after I awoke and
reported that I was first on the list. Initially I thought this to be
good news – no hanging around for hours with nothing to think
about but one's date with destiny. But then I began to consider
other interpretations. Do surgeons need to warm up? Or, even
worse, sober up? What if the chief surgeon was a closet boozer and
had been on a bender the night before? None of us do our best
work while bleary-eyed and with a thumping headache. Perhaps
second on the list would have been better.

I put these worries to one side when Cheryl appeared in the
ward. She had volunteered to pass the info on my likely return time
from the surgery to my mother, who was staying at our house, and
was planning to be by my side when I came round from the anesthetic. As soon as Cheryl, after giving me a suitably reassuring pep
talk on the surgeon's apparently impeccable drinking habits, trotted
off to deliver the timing schedule to Mom, she was replaced at my

bedside by a short, rotund, bald man. This unlikely apparition announced himself as being the hospital barber.

I have to admit that this was a completely unexpected development. I'm not sure I had ever taken notice before of the hairiness of my tummy, and it had never once occurred to me that abdominal surgery would require one to be professionally shaved beforehand. If I was in any doubt as to his veracity (after all, anyone can walk into a hospital with a few props and invent a role for himself, which is a disturbing thought), he immediately opened up his bag and produced what looked to be a professional, if somewhat dated-looking, shaving kit. He pottered off to the sink and returned with a porcelain mug brimming over with shaving foam, brandishing what looked a rather fine example of a badger-hair shaving brush. I was beginning to warm to the idea already, especially when he produced from the bag, not the cut-throat razor I had feared, but a trusty Gillette.

I lay back and stared at the ceiling while he lathered up and then began expertly shaving my tummy. I was quite enjoying the experience, imagining myself to be some overly pampered Roman gladiator on the morning of a big fight, when I heard him mutter "We'd better remove this lot to be on the safe side." Just as my brain was beginning to process his comment, I was shocked to realize that he was now lathering up my pubic hair. This experience had now moved from relaxing to anything but. I closed my eyes and concentrated like never before on remaining perfectly still. This was not the time for an involuntary twitch. He held up my winkie as though inspecting a dubious-looking sausage at the butchers and, in three deft strokes, left me as naked as the day I was born.

Where did he learn this skill? I remember my granddad once telling me that barbers who used cut-throat razors practiced on lathered-up inflated balloons to perfect their art, but I could not fathom how and on what he would have learned this particular aspect of barbering. And who on earth would have been foolish enough to have been his first victim?

My toes uncurling, I was just hugely relieved to have survived the experience intact.

As the barber waddled off to prune his next victim, it seemed we were now in hurry up mode. Sister Grey was next in line, bringing me the usual two open gowns to put on in place of my jimmies. No sooner had I accomplished the task than there appeared a porter pushing a bed on wheels that was to be my carriage to the operating theatre.

No matter how positive and upbeat you are in the run-up to surgery, when you are on the trolley rattling your way to your appointment with the knife, it would be inhuman not to have thoughts of your own mortality go through your mind. As I watched the fluorescent lights pass over my head, I wondered if this would be the last sight I would ever see. Hardly an inspiring one. I can't imagine many poets being moved to greatness by a seemingly endless row of fluorescent lights amid a sea of sickly, institutional green paint. So to avoid any passing of my life before my eyes or mental writing of a new will, I focused on trying to figure out where in the labyrinthine hospital we were heading.

Unlike many patients, I was in full control of my thoughts at this late stage in the process as I was still compos mentis. Because of my obvious upbeat attitude, and the fact that I was first on the list with minimal worrying time, the anesthetist who paid me a flying visit the previous evening had determined that I did not require what's known in the trade as a pre-op, i.e. a sedative, which I was relieved about.

Although it varies by hospital and even by surgeon/anesthetist, you may find yourself under intense pressure to have a pre-op, even if you don't want one. A quick internet search on the subject as I was writing this threw up some scary-sounding responses from medical professionals to someone who asked whether or not one could decline a pre-op. "Every medication your doctor orders for you is in your best interest", "Pre-op sedation is not just a convenience", "You can refuse anything, but your surgeon probably won't like it", "Take the sedative so you will not suffer from anxiety and freak out because that is usually what happens to people like you". You get the picture – it's more for their benefit than yours.

Tip #33: Refuse the Pre-op

I realize that I perhaps am not in the mainstream here as many people about to undergo major surgery would happily strangle someone to ensure they are dosed up to the eyeballs well before the event. I prefer not. Partly because I want to see for myself that the surgeon is not drunk, wild-eyed or suffering from a nervous tic. Also, partly because, right until the administration of the anesthetic, I want to be able to confirm my identity and ensure no operative mix-ups occur. In Britain, one patient a week is listed for the wrong operation and one patient a month gets an operation on the wrong part of their body. Stay awake and make sure you're not the unlucky sod.

I was wheeled towards surgery not at the slovenly pace normally associated with hospital transportation, but at a fast lick. Surgery porters know only too well not to keep the surgeon waiting.

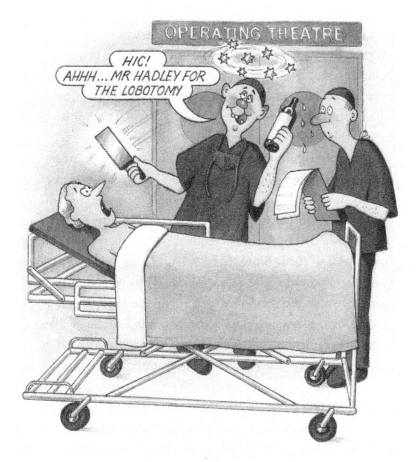

Stay awake, don't nod and dream

Once in the ante-room it was a last check of the name tag on my wrist, a reassuring little pep talk from the surgeon (who thankfully seemed bright as a button) about having a little look around inside, then the anesthetist took over, sending me quickly and expertly into the darkness.

With my previous pile-removal surgical procedure, I seem to recall a very gentle awakening after it was all over. This time, however, it was anything but. My first vague awareness was of incredibly painful abdominal spasms which I later discovered were caused by a tube being inserted into my stomach via the nose and throat. Under normal conditions, such spasms can be very uncomfortable, but when you have just had your abdomen stitched up not ten minutes earlier, the pain is magnified a hundredfold.

As the abdominal spasms subsided, I had the dimmest awareness of someone calling my name and telling me to squeeze their thumb, which I was apparently holding. Then, still at the outer edges of my consciousness, there followed a bumpy ride back to the ward, finished off with an unceremonious and very painful dumping back onto my bed. Now that I wasn't being prodded, poked or tossed around like a side of beef, I could slip back into the netherworld between the conscious and unconscious.

My next awareness was most strange: I could feel my consciousness returning quite quickly but, somewhat alarmingly, I was unable to move, which included even opening my eyes. I could quite clearly hear my mother quizzing Sister Grey on the operation and expected outcome, but was unable to jump in with questions of my own. This state of suspended animation moved from alarming to frustrating as, throughout what was becoming a prolonged conversation, Mom was rubbing my hand with a motherly tenderness. Only to me, being unable to move a muscle, it soon turned into a version of the Chinese water torture where, even though the motion was gentle enough, the unstoppable repetitiveness was beginning to drive me nuts.

Even today, with all the modern technology at their fingertips, the medical profession struggles to accept that patients are never anything other than either unconscious or awake, even though many patients describe the same kind of phenomenon as happened to me. This effect of being wide awake while seeming comatose to by-standers is brought about by the fact that when you have a general anesthetic for an operation, you don't just have an anesthetic.

The first modern-day anesthetic, nitrous oxide (laughing gas), was discovered at the turn of the 18th-century by Sir Humphry Davy; a remarkable man who also discovered many elements (e.g. calcium, sodium and potassium), not to mention inventing the miners safety lamp that bears his name. Although nitrous oxide cannot induce unconsciousness, it is still used to this day to help keep you under. As well as not being the ideal knock-out gas, a further limitation in its use became apparent in its first public demonstration for painless tooth extraction when the patient yelled the place down.

This phenomenon, that anesthetics do not provide pain relief, applies to most unconsciousness-inducing gases in use today where intense pain encountered during a surgical procedure has the potential to wake you up. To counteract this, in addition to an anesthetic you are given an analgesic to dull the pain. The third component of the general anesthetic process is a muscle relaxant to overcome the body's natural inclination to go into spasm when you are being cut open and having your key components yanked about. This is derived from curare, a substance used by Amazonian tribes on the tips of their blow-darts to paralyze their prey. You have no guarantee that each of these three components of general anesthesia will wear off at exactly the same rate. What had happened in my case was that the muscle relaxant was wearing off more slowly than the anesthetic itself, so I was waking up, but immobile.

However, I gradually regained the use of my muscles and gave everyone the impression of waking up an hour later than I actually did. By this time, Cheryl had reappeared with some stunning news.

She had received a phone call soon after the start of my operation, instructing her to bring her camera to one of the operating theatres, as the surgeon wanted some photographs taken of his handiwork. This was a common occurrence in Cheryl's workday, although in this instance she approached the suite of operating theatres with some trepidation knowing that I was in one of them.

Her trepidation turned out to be justified as she had indeed been summoned by my surgeon. Completely unbeknownst to me beforehand, this surgeon was not a local hacker, but was actually one of the leading lights globally in the surgical treatment of Inflammatory Bowel diseases. Even more amazingly, he had invented a brand new technique for dealing with my particular problem – strictures – and had decided to use this innovation on me for only the third time ever. Since my strictures were such classic examples, he wanted to have Cheryl photograph the process for future teaching and publication.

Obviously this put Cheryl in a dilemma. It's one thing taking pictures of some portion of anatomy while having no idea who it is lying underneath the swathe of green, sterile sheets, but quite another doing so when you know full well it's a friend of yours under there. Apparently, quite a debate ensued between Cheryl and the surgeon as to whether this was a good idea, but she bravely pressed on, put personal feelings aside and did her duty.

Two interesting features came out of Cheryl having been present and snapping away during my operation. While we were chatting, I related to her two memories that were quite clear in my mind that must have come from when I was just going under or just coming around. The first was briefly seeing a multi-bulbed and extremely bright bank of lights overhead, and the second was a brief snatch of conversation I had heard that went something like, "Well this has never happened before."

Cheryl's eyes popped out of her head and her jaw went crashing to the floor as though in a Tom and Jerry cartoon. Firstly, she said, with this surgeon, the patient is anaesthetized and brought round not in the theatre itself, but in an ante-room which has just normal strip-lighting, so the lights I described could only have been those in the operating theatre itself where I was supposed to be fully anaesthetized. And secondly, the conversation I had heard, and that Cheryl had personally witnessed, occurred not at the beginning or end, but right in the middle of what had been a four-hour operation. What had happened was that they had been forced to halt the operation as I had developed a case of hiccoughs, a situation never previously encountered by the surgeon.

Cheryl quizzed me fiercely as to was I sure that no one had told me this after my being returned to the ward and that perhaps I was just mistaking it for a memory? But, at this stage, the surgical team was still in theatre dealing with the rest of its day's operating list; I had not seen anyone who had been in there apart from Cheryl herself. What this meant, in conjunction with seeing the operating lights overhead, was that I had briefly come round during the operation when I was split open from breastbone to pubis with half my insides splayed out on my abdomen. Eeeek!

Internet research suggests that this occurs in up to one percent of all surgical procedures, but how reliable is this statistic? If Cheryl hadn't been in there it is highly unlikely I would have mentioned it to anyone; after all, when it happened I was not aware that the operation was underway. If it's one percent of patients who are FULLY aware at some stage during an operation then there must be many more who become briefly aware and then either forget about it (anesthesia induces partial amnesia) or put it down as a dream.

The reality is that the danger with anesthetic is not that you will never wake up again, but that you might partially wake up halfway through. You are kept just bubbling under the state of consciousness rather than on the brink of death, mainly because too much anesthesia can result in vomiting upon awakening, which is less than desirable when you have just had dozens of stitches in your abdomen, so I'm not complaining.

Tip #34: The Best Surgeons Use the Best Anesthetists

As a rule of thumb, the better surgeons will make sure they only work with the better anesthetists so as not to have their batting averages brought down by an anesthetist who dozes off at the controls. It's another reason to get yourself in with the best surgeon you can find – you double your chances of not having your life in the hands of an incompetent idiot.

At the end of this momentous day, I was honored with the appearance of the second-in-command of the surgical team who had come along to give us the post-match report. He related that there had been two different elements to my surgery. The bleeding from my university days, which had returned in the few months leading up to the operation, had been the first symptom to be addressed. The source of the blood loss was a foot-long section of small bowel, just where it attaches to the large bowel, which was extremely diseased and inflamed as to be almost permanently oozing blood. The only solution for this had been to remove the entire inflamed section, along with my appendix (another organ I'd apparently be better off without), together with the valve that acts as the boundary between the two bowels.

The second phase of the operation had been to fix three strictures that had been the source of the mega-painful abdominal gripes, which lay much further upstream. Prior to my surgeon's invention of his revolutionary technique – christened a strictureplasty – the only treatment had been to remove the portion of bowel in which the stricture lay, then join the two ends together. The trouble with this approach is that if you developed a lot of strictures, you could very quickly run out of small bowel and be unable to maintain adequate nutrition via eating and drinking. In fact I had noticed several patients to whom this had happened who came into the ward two or three times a week to spend a couple of hours hooked up to a machine being intravenously fed.

The new approach was designed to preserve precious bowel by widening the narrowed area rather than removing it. The technique itself, like most surgery from what I can see, was really nothing more than the most basic plumbing technique. I am surprised that surgeons don't operate with the crack in their butt in full view. Maybe they do under that flowing gown – who knows?

The technique in my case began with a small incision at the top end of the small bowel, enabling the insertion of a device specially designed to find the strictures which are invisible when looking at the bowel from the outside. This gizmo is basically a small inflatable balloon on the end of a flexible long ruler. The balloon is inserted into the small bowel and pushed along until it gets stuck at a stricture, with the calibration on the flexible ruler attachment telling the surgeon how far along the bowel lies the stricture. The ball can be inflated to whatever diameter the surgeon requires, based on how radical he wants to be in determining how many and what kind of strictures he wants to address. In my case, the ball was only modestly inflated so that it would only get stuck at any strictures that were quite bad and most likely to be getting blocked on a frequent basis.

Knowing the location of the first stricture, the surgeon then opens up the bowel at that point with a cut of about three inches along its length. The two sides of this cut are pulled apart as far as possible until the two ends of the cut meet in the middle. The tissue is then sewn up at right angles to the length of the bowel creating, in effect, a right angle in the direction of the bowel that is, even with the inflamed tissue of the stricture still in place, a significantly wider diameter than normal bowel, thus enabling partly digested food to pass through without hindrance. The balloon is then pushed further along until the next roadblock and so on until the end of the small bowel is reached.

The insight behind this brilliantly simple technique is that the food getting stuck and causing massive pain is much more of a problem to the patient than the fact that the bowel tissue is inflamed, and that any symptoms from the inflammation itself are worth putting up with rather than losing precious bowel length. Previous research had shown that patients who had strictures removed were just as likely to develop new ones as patients who had them left in situ, so there was no real downside to leaving the tissue in place as long as the narrowing was dealt with.

These days, given the much greater concerns over disgruntled patients taking legal action, it would be unthinkable that you would be given as sketchy an advance briefing as I had received. But it could well be the case that the surgeon has only the haziest idea of what he will find while rooting around inside you. Once he finds the problem, he can hardly wake you up to ask you to sign a permission form for a specific procedure, so beforehand you are usually asked to sign what amounts to a blank check.

Tip #35: Find Out What You Are Letting Yourself in For

Well before the event, do as much quizzing as you can of the specialist who is referring you for the operation on what are the most common issues and procedures with your kind of surgery. Then you can go and do your research beforehand.

In my case, because the technique was so new, any pre-research on strictureplasties would have been a waste of time. This raises the next question: Should you sign up for new and innovative treatments? Obviously, it is tempting to let them practice on other people until they have figured out all the kinks, but then you could be missing out on a life-changing improvement. If everyone adopted the wait-and-see approach, we'd still be having legs amputated in twenty seconds flat while clenching our teeth on a leather strap.

Tip #36: Leading Edge or Bleeding Edge?

If it's an established technique, ask how many that particular surgeon has done and his success rate. If it's a novel technique, find out how well respected in the particular specialty he is. Thanks to the internet, I now see my surgeon's name quoted in numerous academic papers and in conference presentations. Had I known that at the time, it would have given me the confidence to sign up to be the third one in. On the other hand, if he was an unknown, forget it. I have never come across a self-doubting surgeon, so just because he is planning to do something doesn't automatically mean he will be competent at it.

I asked if it would be possible for me to have a copy of Cheryl's photographs, which apparently showed this technique in all its glory. My request met with an immediate and definite refusal – the surgeon was concerned how I would react emotionally to seeing my insides laid out like the offal section of the butcher's counter. But I persisted as, right from when I had first ventured into Birmingham Central Library, I had been a firm believer in that the more I knew about what was happening to me, both medically and surgically, the better able to positively influence events I would be. After a couple of days, the medics relented and I was given a copy and treated to a blow-by-blow account of the technique. I still have these photographs today and I believe that one or two of them did indeed make it into a medical textbook. Fame at last!

Tip #37: Say Cheese

Unless you are good friends with a hospital's medical illustrator, you are unlikely to get a set of snapshots of your surgery. But there are now many medical investigative procedures that produce images. Personally, I found every image helpful in taking ownership of my Crohn's, but it may not be for you. If you start collecting them, be more circumspect than was I in whipping them out and passing them around at tea-parties with friends and relatives. A small minority claim never to have slept well since.

The punch line of the operation debriefing was that, once recovered from the surgery itself, I would feel better than I had for years, which was music to my ears. But what I wasn't told was just how traumatic the simple-sounding process of "recovering" would be, and just how short-lived would be the period of feeling better. At this stage, it had not yet sunk in with me that, while operations could help alleviate symptoms, they could do nothing to alter the inexorable course of what was and is an incurable condition.

Getting Better All The Time

"The patient must minister to himself."

— Shakespeare (Macbeth, Act 5, Scene 3)

AFTER ALL THE excitement of the day, the euphoria of actually surviving the operation and being the centre of attention for the first few hours after coming round, the grim reality of recovering from major surgery began to set in during the night. Of course, it stood to reason that the aftermath of being sliced open and having my insides yanked about for several hours might not be completely painless. Millions of nerve fibers had been severed and wouldn't be doing their job properly if they did not register some protest, but I had no idea just how much they would do so.

As I lay on my back, I could barely move any muscle more than a fraction without triggering an unbelievably intense pain spasm in my abdomen. I weakly pressed the call button that had been placed in my hand and, once answered by one of the nursing night shift, I enquired as to the available pain relief options. They were disappointingly few. To ease the intensity of the spasms, I could have the use of a small electric heating pad that could be placed on top of my incision site, which was the source of the worst pain. While it certainly helped and the warmth felt somewhat comforting, it was barely making a dent on the real pain. The surgical aftermath was proving to be so intense as to make me question why I had signed up for surgery to treat symptoms that seemed so trivial in comparison to what I was now enduring.

I have found this to be a common feature of all my subsequent surgeries. You go into it feeling that you would do absolutely anything to address your symptoms, yet, in the first twenty-four hours post-operation, you feel such a weakling for having succumbed to the siren-call of surgery when the agony you now suffer seems a hundred times worse than had been the symptoms. Surely I could have held out if I had known it was going to be like this.

Tip #38: Put Surgery Off, But Not Indefinitely

When you reach the stage of being convinced you need major surgery to address your symptoms, steel yourself to put it off for another six months. Crohn's is an illness of slow degeneration, so nothing will happen that is likely to kill you. Whereas surgery and anesthesia can kill you, plus the recovery is invariably a much bigger ordeal than you fondly imagine from that portrayed in medical dramas.

The only other weapon in the pain relief locker was to have injections of morphine. As this was taking place in 1983, the technology in administering the drug was a somewhat unsophisticated injection into my thigh every three hours. Having these morphine shots was the most bittersweet experience of my life. The sweet component was that it undoubtedly did what it said on the box and dulled the pain to tolerable levels, but the bitterness was manifold. Firstly, the real pain relief lasted for well under an hour before it began to wear off, making the next two hours seem like a lifetime as I watched the clock tick round with a ridiculous slowness until I could have my next shot. Is this how heroin addicts feel? It's made from the same stuff after all.

When it finally came time for the next shot, the lead night nurse and a nursing assistant would assemble by my bed and the one would religiously recite my name and hospital number from my wristband to be confirmed by the other that I was the intended recipient. So welcome was this ritual that my hospital number,

414322, will be forever etched on my mind as being the signal of imminent relief from the unendurable.

But the relief from pain did not come free of charge; in fact, I soon began to wonder if it was worth the price I was paying. Almost immediately on receiving the injection, I would fall asleep but be subject to the most terrifying and intense nightmares from which I would thankfully awaken only to find that I had been asleep for maybe three or four minutes. I became too scared to go back to sleep, thus prolonging an exhaustion that was doing nothing to help me feel any better. When the drug was working, the more likely I was to fall asleep and be terrified out of my wits; as the drug wore off, the nightmares lessened but the pain increased. This first night would have been rejected by Edgar Allan Poe as a horror story too unbelievable to tell. Subject me to The Pit and the Pendulum anytime; it was the longest and worst night of my life.

Mine was by no means an uncommon reaction to morphine; the dreams can verge on being hallucinations. Things have improved in that, these days, you don't have to wait hours for the next shot as it is now administered either by an automatic pump or by the patient pressing a button to activate a measured dose. In both cases you have some control over the amount given, but morphine is still morphine.

Tip #39: Stay Off the Drugs as Much as You Can

Allow yourself only the minimum amount necessary to take the pain level to something you can just about endure. Bearing pain is not as bad as the nightmares.

Finally, the night passed and life began to return to the ward. With things going on to distract me, I found I could bear the pain for longer and not have the morphine so frequently. But just as I was feeling relieved, the medical profession found other diabolical ways to torment me.

First up was the physiotherapist, a jovial, stout girl who, on the face of it, was not the best advert for exercise I had ever seen. However, it turned out that she needed all her bulk for the heavy lifting that her job entailed. Since I professed myself completely incapable of wriggling up the bed to sit in a more upright position, she leant over, grasped me under both armpits and yanked me up in one easy for her but exquisitely painful moment for me. However, the pain was compensated for by my head being plunged into her matronly bosom, giving me a fleeting sample of Helen Keller's life of being simultaneously rendered dumb, blind and deaf as I was enveloped in her décolletage.

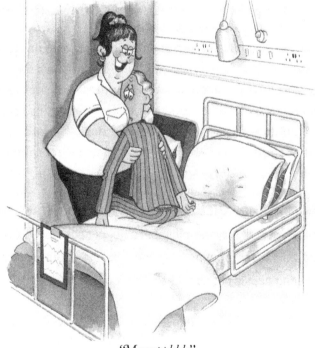

"Mmmpphhh"

As she pulled away and I could breathe once more, she launched into the real reason for her visit: instructing me on the need to have a good cough once an hour. This was necessary because the combined effects of a prolonged bout of anesthesia and being immobile on one's back could easily lead to the accumulation of fluid in the lungs, which could have all kinds of unwelcome ramifications, including death from pneumonia. Having successfully got my attention, she demonstrated the kind of cough she was looking for. And what a cough it was. It began with a deep rumble that seemed to start in her all-too-sensible shoes, which then increased in volume like the approach of a deadly avalanche, culminating in a lung-busting phlegm-remover the likes of which would have made a 60-a-day smoker feel that perhaps they should be cutting back a bit.

While my ward-mates who congregated for endless cigarettes in the television room could have perhaps made a decent effort at matching her, my first attempt was so pathetically weak that she was by no means sure I had actually yet tried to follow her lead. Even after much coaching and cajoling, because of the pain from my incision site, the best I could manage was the kind of barely-audible discreet cough by which a sommelier would announce his presence at your table.

Since this was better than nothing, she then moved on to the next task which, much to my horror, was that she was going to help me get out of bed and sit in the bedside armchair. I could not believe my ears. Here I was, weak as a kitten and unable even to muster a half-decent cough, and I was going to have to stand up and walk over to the chair? But my protests fell on deaf ears; we were going to do it whether I thought I could or not. I find it amazing in hindsight just how cowed and obedient I'm made by the young girls who run hospital wards. Is it the uniforms?

Tip #40: Let the Kids Boss You Around

While, as you may have gathered, I am not a fan of slavishly hanging onto every word the doctor says, I advocate doing just that with the other professions who make up the medical team. Nurses, physiotherapists, phlebotomists (the people who take your blood), dieticians and so on all seem to know exactly what they are doing and never once have I suffered by meekly going along with their wishes.

With another dose of breast-envelopment, which I suspect she knowingly used as both encouragement and sound-dampening, we got myself sat up on the side of the bed after a good five minutes of her grunting and my uttering heavily muffled protests of pain. At this point we paused while the waves of agony gently ebbed back to bearability. In addition to the pain from the incision site, there were the strangest sensations from inside my abdomen: it seemed like all the parts which had been yanked about were slithering back to their normal positions or that my nightmare of having swallowed snakes was, in fact, a repressed memory and had really happened.

Then came the moment of truth in that I now had to stand up and shuffle over to the chair. To help with this seemingly impossible maneuver, she grasped me in a bear hug and did most of the lifting such that my feet were merely brushing the ground. She then let me down onto my feet ever so gently, ignoring my increasingly shrill squeals as I took more and more of my own weight. After another pause to again let the pain diminish, she then assisted me in shuffling over to the chair at a snail's pace, held me in the by now familiar semi-suffocation pose and lowered me into the armchair that she had helpfully padded with a brace of pillows.

I would never have expected getting from a bed to an adjacent chair would class as a major success in my life, but once there I had a euphoric sense of achievement. There is no way on earth I would have thought it possible to do what we had just done and, if it had been down to me, I wouldn't even have contemplated trying. It is important to recognize when you have your first surgery that, while you are a complete novice and enduring situations and pain levels beyond your past experiences, you are surrounded by professionals who have seen it all before.

Tip #41: Enjoy the Early Achievements

Suspend your natural reluctance to curl up amidst your misery and you will surprise yourself with your body's own capabilities.

Now that I was actually mobile, I made the switch from chair to bed and back again several times that day entirely under my own steam, each journey being slightly less traumatic than the last. I took great pleasure in being sat in the chair when both Cheryl and Mom came to visit during the day, seeing the genuine surprise in their expressions. The same was not the case, however, with my other visitors who were all seeing me post-operatively for the first time and were clearly shocked to the core by my emaciated appearance. But a steady stream of visitors is good for one's morale and punctuates what are otherwise very long and featureless days.

One feature I noticed from having colleagues come visiting, was just how completely disinterested I had become in their work conversations. It all seemed so pathetically trite and irrelevant compared to the life-changing experience of just having undergone major surgery. I soon found it a good idea to ask no questions whatsoever about what had been going on in the office in my absence; indeed to contribute as little as possible as talking was incredibly tiring. On a more positive note, it was very gratifying to see the number of cards one received and the humor contained within. Madeleine, who was away on a long assignment during this whole process, thoughtfully included in her card the somewhat puzzling advice to refrain from spitting grape pips down the toilet as she had been scolded for doing so on her one and only hospitalization years ago.

Back to my recovery, there were two events of note, both revolving around the fact that, after a general anesthetic, not all the parts of your body spring back to life at the same rate. The bowels, which normally coax your food along with their slow, wave-like motion known as peristalsis, are rendered comatose by anesthesia, and even more so when they have been manhandled during surgery, as mine had been. Because of this, together with the stitching up of my recently severed small bowel, there was obviously no chance of me having anything to eat for a while, so I was being kept alive through the drip that was affixed to my arm.

As my kidneys were already up and running, all this extra fluid entering my system was being filtered out and sent down to the bladder. Unfortunately the bladder itself was also paralyzed following anesthesia, so, during the day, I was feeling more and more desperate for a pee. However, every time I asked for one of those papier mache pee bottles, I was frustratingly unable to perform. Not knowing at the time that paralysis was the problem, I assumed that by propping myself up as far on my side as possible, I could get gravity working in my favor, but to no avail. Every couple of hours a nurse would come round, update my fluids chart which kept a record of the quantity going in, tut loudly and ask with decreasing patience if I had managed to pee. It was like being back in the first year of elementary school.

By early evening, she was muttering dark threats. If I continued to let her down, she would have to insert a catheter to do the job for me before I got fluid overload. Several of my ward-mates were toting catheter bags, so I knew she wasn't bluffing. Also working in her favor was the fact that, from where I was lying, here was another medical procedure that sounded like it would be much better conducted while under general anesthetic. The thought of being a wide-awake, passive participant in the insertion of an improbably large and unyielding plastic tube into a depressingly small and blancmange-like organ was too much to bear. My trepidation was even higher than would normally be expected by this threat due to the anesthesia seeming to have had the same effect on my twinkie as when going for a swim off the boardwalk in Atlantic City. Peeled shrimp would be the best description of the current state of my manhood.

Such was my motivation to avoid the catheter that I spent the next three hours with my willie inside the pee bottle willing, through force of thought, the deluge to begin. To supplement the mind over matter, I adopted every feasible position to enroll the help of gravity within the limitations of the still eye-watering pain in my abdomen. Even though I was conducting all my efforts under the bedclothes, I could see that I was raising a few eyebrows from the visitors who were now trickling into the ward, who were clearly misinterpreting the grunting, groaning and obvious manipulation going on around my groin area.

Hospital wards, by their very nature, do not afford you the levels of privacy you are probably used to. So it can be easy to allow your natural modesty to prevail over the need to address a problem with some bodily function or other, especially when the wife of the man in the next bed is clearly peeking over her knitting.

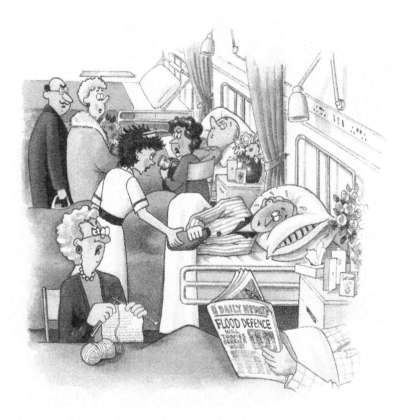

Privates on parade

Tip #42: Just Do It

Sometimes you just have to put normal standards aside and get on with whatever you need to do without worrying about frightening the horses or making yourself liable for a charge of indecent exposure. Never forget that hospitals are for the benefit of the patients. Crohn's is an illness where the main symptoms involve things best left out of polite conversation, so if you can't put your management of its symptoms first in a hospital, then where can you?

Just when it felt like my bladder was about to explode, my efforts paid off with what was the most satisfying pee of my life, the only problem then being that, once the dam had been breached, the flow was seemingly endless. In a panic, as the bottle was rapidly approaching full capacity and there seemed to be no way I could stem the flow, I hailed a passing 1-stripe student nurse and pleaded for a second pee receptacle. She returned just in time and I was able, with her help, to make the switch without any significant spillage; this being important as she had to record the volume coming out and calibrate with the records of the volume that had gone in. Thankfully, this was the last drama of the day, although I knew it would be followed by another night of nightmare-filled, intermittent sleep punctuated by pain-filled waits for the next dose of morphine.

As the next day dawned, my successes the previous day of making it to the bedside chair and foiling the catheter threat kicked in my competitive streak and inspired me to treat this immediate recovery period as a challenge to be conquered. I began by quizzing the nurses and then the more junior members of the surgical team who wandered by on what were the norms with this kind of surgery for patients being up and mobile, eating and ultimately being discharged home. The answers to each question I saw as a target to be smashed. My new go-getting attitude would be immediately put to the test with the news that, unlike the previous day when I had had the dubious privilege of a bed bath, today I would be having a shower.

My initial excitement at this new challenge was tempered by the twin realization that, a) the shower room was at the far end of the ward and thus would involve at least twenty times the walking that I had done so far, and b) that the pretty student nurse who had been assigned this task was apparently going to be in there with me (ooo-err!) as there was no way I would be able to, for example, reach down and wash my feet. Thankfully, unlike during some of my earlier medical tests, erection-phobia was the farthest thing from my mind as it was by now clear that anesthesia-induced paralysis was in full swing in that department, there being no circumstances imaginable where the peeled prawn would spring to life.

Clutching my drip stand with the one hand and the nurse with the other, I set off on the journey that seemed as daunting to me as must have the trek to the North Pole for Admiral Peary. Each painful shuffle of the feet seemed to take me no nearer my goal, and we had to stop several times for me to recover enough strength to continue. We eventually got there and I had a more than welcome sit-down while the nurse taped a plastic bag over my incision site that was still, at this stage, covered by the blood-stained dressing that had been applied immediately I had been sewn up.

The logistics of showering in my condition were that, after completely disrobing – a task greatly complicated by every movement being painful and there being a drip in my arm – I shuffled over to another chair that lay in line of fire of the shower nozzle. I sat and appreciated the warm, refreshing shower while she did most of the hard work. Although she had given me a good, soapy scrubbing elsewhere, the one concession to my modesty was she handed me the facecloth for "my bits".

After another painfully slow walk back to the bed, punctuated by numerous rest stops, I flopped into my chair exhilarated by the achievement. Over the next couple of days, I strove to do more and more walks, going further and further afield each time. I was able to shower myself, though not as vigorously as had been the case pre the operation, and my coughing was now a quite respectable lung-clearer audible at thirty paces. I had weaned myself off the morphine and everyone seemed both impressed and delighted at the pace of my recovery.

On the dietary side, nothing had been allowed to pass my lips by this time as there had not yet been any evidence that the bowels had recovered their powers of motion, the first sign of which would be the passing of wind. By Day 4 after the operation, I was being quizzed almost on an hourly basis as to whether or not I had farted, though for once not in usual accusatory sense of: "Was it YOU who farted?"

The first evidence that things are stirring comes not with a fart but with the feeling of wind moving around your system. A bit like with the urine, things have to build up almost to bursting point before the muscles at the far end of the system begrudgingly return into action. Consequently, I spent a full day and night suffering from increasingly painful built-up wind that, when reaching its greatest intensity, manifested itself not as abdominal discomfort but as a really painful ache in the left shoulder – who would have guessed? I even resorted to requesting some of the dreaded morphine during the night to relieve this new pain which, at that stage, I had no idea was related to the wind build-up.

Late into the night, I did the tiniest of farts that was so insubstantial I wasn't sure myself that it had indeed been one. But having accomplished the feat once, the system was soon in full throttle, passing prolonged raspers powerful enough to set my bed sheets flapping. Interestingly, for any fart connoisseurs, they were completely odorless, a feature I later discovered was due to the total absence of bacteria in my system; as an addition to my diet of saline drip, there had also been regular doses of super-powerful intravenous antibiotics.

Now things were working again – a piece of news that had been greeted by a burst of applause from the surgical team who visited during their morning rounds – I could begin to be reintroduced to what were for me the long-forgotten pleasures of eating and drinking. Prior to the first sip of water passing my lips, on one of my longer walks, I weighed myself on the scales in Doctor Ray's office so that I could officially record the low point, it being a frighteningly lightweight 118 pounds; hardly surprising since I now hadn't eaten a morsel for over a week.

The way the dietary reintroduction worked was that I began with a thimble-full of water every hour. If, after a full day of this, nothing seemed to have gone amiss, things were gradually stepped up over the next forty-eight hours via cups of tea, jelly and egg custard to the point where I was allowed to have a bowl of cereal for breakfast, followed by a small sandwich for lunch. As real food was now going into the system, there was as much anticipation towards my first bowel movement as had been the case for my peeing and farting.

This being a ward primarily devoted to problems with the bowels, there was a system in place for the inspection of everyone's bowel movements, which was revealed to me as the time for my first one came close. Every poop had to be done into a bed pan, which the pooper then placed into a large paper bag upon which they wrote their name and time of pooping. Several times a day, the student nurse who had drawn the short straw would have the job of inspecting each effort and then grading it accordingly, recording weight, consistency and so on in the patient's notes.

As the day went on, I could feel things stirring and, when I thought action seemed imminent, armed myself with a crossword and pen and tottered off to the toilet. Much to my surprise, since the runs had been an increasingly frequent feature of my life in the months prior to the operation, I had almost finished the cryptic crossword before the turtle gradually appeared from its shell. Once out however, it was followed by quite a landslide. As I stood up and bent down to pick up the bed pan in order to follow the prescribed recording process, I knew instantly that all was not well.

Firstly, I was feeling quite lightheaded, which I could have attributed to the elation of passing my first motion if I had not seen that the bedpan was filled, not with a humdinger of a floater, but with a series of black bullets swimming in an inky, crude oil-like fluid. I gamely managed to fill in the details on the paper bag and put the bed-pan on the shelf before leaving the toilet and promptly fainting into the arms of a student nurse who had noticed that I was looking a lot worse than when I had gone in thirty minutes earlier.

I came to amidst what seemed like barely-controlled pandemonium around my bed. My saline drip had been replaced by a bag of blood, the contents of which were snaking its way down the tube towards my vein while I was simultaneously having an injection into my other arm. This I learnt later was Vitamin K given to quickly stop bleeding. A couple of work colleagues from Cadbury's turned up at this point to visit and were promptly ushered away as the curtains were pulled round my bed.

By this stage I was in a complete shock and panic, assuming that the surgery had gone horribly wrong and that I was either going to bleed to death there and then or, almost as frightening for me, was going to be taken back into the operating theatre and have to undergo not only more surgery but what had been a barely endurable post-operative recovery. I needed a friendly face at this point and, as Mom had already been and gone by then, I asked a nurse to phone Cheryl, who worked in the building, requesting that she come ASAP. She rushed in five minutes later when, for the first time in at least a decade, I promptly burst into tears such was my fear of what the immediate future held.

Having to calm a blubbing flat-mate is, I think, above and beyond the call of duty, but Cheryl didn't flinch and did a marvelous job of reassuring me. Once I was reasonably composed, she went off to quiz the second-in-command of the surgical team who had been busy inspecting the contents of my bed pan. He came back with her and, in my opinion, gave me a complete whitewash about how a bit of blood can accumulate in the bowel during the surgery and that this was what, most likely, had made its way out. I don't know if he really expected me to fall for such a thin storyline as it bore no relation to the mass of activity that had preceded it, but, as I was feeling a bit brighter, I let it pass.

The aftermath to this frightening event came from an unexpected quarter. When all had calmed down and everyone gone back to their normal duties, a patient from the other end of the ward came over and sat beside my bed. We had not talked together at all until this point in my stay, so he introduced himself and asked if I minded him passing on a bit of advice. Not at all.

He explained he was in the hospital for some long-running liver complaint and that he had been watching my slogging around the place in my quest to be the fastest recoverer ever. This, he advised me, was a big mistake. Not so much the slogging, but the mindset that I could and should "beat" my condition. He went on to explain his philosophy about coping with long-term illness. I forget his exact words, but I have never forgotten the message.

Firstly, it's most likely going to be for the rest of your life so, by definition, you cannot beat it – it will always be there. This then means that you should not try to live your life exactly as it was before you were ill. That life is gone now. But that doesn't mean you just give up and become a victim, because then you will lose control over the direction of your new life to the vagaries of your illness. It's about give and take. Sometimes you can live life as you would have done before, but there are other times where you must give precedence to your illness.

Rather than resting as much as possible and giving my body the opportunity to repair itself, I had been treating the surgery as a challenge to be overcome, rather like playing through a muscle injury to keep my place in the football team. While that may work for a temporary condition, if I kept doing it for the rest of my life then, at some point, I would come badly unstuck, as I seem to have nearly done with this episode.

Contracting a chronic illness such as Crohn's is a life-changing event. You encounter many novel situations and circumstances having not only had no warning, but probably never given a moment's thought to what life with illness must be like. However, countless people have trodden the same path, so you would be foolish not to learn from their experiences whenever you can.

Tip #43: Learn From Those Around You

Hospitals are universities of living with illness, so it's another reason not to lock yourself away in a private room where you cannot observe and learn from other people's coping techniques.

Given the profound impact this man would have on my life, you'd think I could at least remember his name, but I can't. But better that than forget his message, because it is the foundation stone of how to be successful at being ill with Crohn's, and was advice that I would begin to apply from that day forwards.

Boulevard Of Broken Dreams

"Great effort is required to arrest decay and restore vigor. One must exercise proper deliberation, plan carefully before making a move, and be alert in guarding against relapse following a renaissance."

— Horace (65BC – 8BC)

I TOOK THE mystery liver patient's advice to heart and spent the remainder of my time in Ward 8, not charging up and down flights of stairs to build back my strength, but resting as much as possible while following to the letter the instructions of an ever-changing cohort of physiotherapists. It seemed that the sturdy, bosomy one was detailed to do her smothering trick with the immobile patients, the follow-up work being done by her more willowy colleagues.

There were times I would awaken feeling as full of energy as a coiled spring, and it was very difficult just to lie on the bed or sit in my chair all day apart from taking a shower and walking my visitors to the ward doors. But I resolved to do it, or perhaps I should say, not do it.

Tip #44: Do Less

Get in some good books and DVD's and consciously do less than you feel capable of doing. Your body is working overtime in repairing the damage done internally, so exercise, especially when you are barely eating yet, merely diverts precious stores of energy away from the main priority and hence is counter-productive.

Thankfully, my recovery continued event-free; I was able to eat increasing amounts and my bowels miraculously recovered, working more normally than they had since my early days at university. The first sign of real progress was my de-coupling from the drip that had kept me alive these past several days. It had almost become a part of me and one that I had an obsessive interest in. If I detected any air bubble inching its way down the tube towards my vein I would go into a minor panic having read somewhere that air bubbles in the bloodstream can kill you. I would frantically flick the tube with my finger to send the bubble back upstream again. Every now and again, I had to prevail on one of the student nurses to come and do the job properly. Being students, I don't think they had been taught yet a fact I only learnt quite recently: that small bubbles are harmless and that it requires the forcible injection of a good syringe-full of air to actually kill you. Indeed, any death by air embolism through an intravenous tube is automatically treated as suspected murder.

The uncovering of my incision site was the next, much anticipated event signaling my recovery. It had been covered by the same adhesive dressing for the entire time since the surgery and I was eagerly looking forward to being able to have a proper shower without the hassle of taping a plastic bag over the site. The removal itself was a painstaking affair, being done a fraction of an inch at a time so as not to open up any bleeding. Once off, I was amazed at the sight. Firstly, the wound itself was much larger than I had expected, starting dead centre on a level with the bottom of my ribcage, running down to the belly button, around which it did a graceful semi-circle, before resuming its central path down to just north of where my pubic hair would have been had it not been shorn off. Apparently, the line down the centre is a favored surgical entry point as it contains few vital nerves and blood vessels.

Given such a large wound, I would have expected there to be dozens of neat stitches to be in place but was shocked to see there were just six. SIX!!! That was one for every two inches of incision! I hardly dared breathe in case I snapped open what seemed to me to be a wholly inadequate means of holding in the Bradley innards.

However, my panic abated when the nurse informed me that all the serious stitching work was actually under the skin, there being several different layers of embroidery holding together the various strata that made up my abdominal wall. Even so, I had expected a higher quality of needlework to be on view than what looked like a completely haphazard beginner's attempt. Mailbags sewn by prisoners would have put this to shame. Instead of anticipating a graceful scar that I could perhaps pass off as having been inflicted in an Olympic fencing competition, it looked like I was destined to be horribly deformed, the surgeon apparently having used a sharpened stick and a pickaxe.

Of course, stitching you up is too menial a task for the head surgeon, who has usually sneaked off for a restorative cigarette by the time your outer layers are being sewn back together. Sewing you up is only one step up the surgical training ladder from holding the suction tube, so your eventual outer appearance is in the hands of someone quite a way down the chain of command.

Tip #45: Plead Beforehand Rather Than Complain Afterwards

If you are at all concerned beforehand about your scar, be sure to let them know before you go under the anesthetic. To increase your chances, log in your concerns about scarring with the person who will actually be stitching you up. They will probably ignore you, but you might get lucky.

I suppose I could have complained about it during the daily rounds of the surgical team, but that would have meant breaking the rules. As the patient, you are allocated a walk-on role only, such as having your belly felt by several clammy-palmed students. The medics do their usual routine of talking about you as though you are not there. On the rare occasion you are asked a question, it comes with the answer already attached, "How are you feeling today Mr. Bradley? Much better I expect without that nasty inflammation inside you!" Just as you are formulating your own answer they are already marching off towards the next bed. The post-operative morning rounds are not a productive environment for you to be able to influence events.

On the morning of Day 7 after the operation, the usual bed-side rounds procedure took a new turn when the head surgeon himself, who usually gave these events a miss, not only graced us all with his presence but announced that I was well enough to be discharged the next day. Plucking up my courage to breach the no-talking rule, I loudly cleared my throat to interrupt his latest medical witticism to the throng, and followed up in the momentary pause to ask what for me was a key question that had been increasingly playing on my mind.

"What is the outlook for me over the foreseeable future?" As the answer was directed to the several students rather than me, it wasn't quite the detailed life-map that I was hoping to hear.

"Strictures do reoccur in a high percentage of patients, so we can expect him to come in every five years or so for a few stricture-plasties." And that was it; off they sallied to discuss the next medical exhibit a few beds down the ward.

With this information, thankfully augmented by the research I had done in Birmingham Central Library, I could at least make a start in beginning to plan my future life. This would now be in partnership, not just with the illness itself, but also with what potentially looked like quite a few repeats of the previous two weeks' trauma followed by prolonged recuperations. Prior to planning the long term, though, the short term of where I was to continue my recovery had to be addressed.

There were only two possible options: the shared house in Birmingham or back in the parental nest up in Lancashire. The choice was clear, especially to my mother. Even though I was feeling better each day, I was still basically doing nothing so going back to my parents' place for a while seemed the best option. Both were at home all day and could fetch cups of tea on demand. Plus, of course, Mom was an experienced nurse. Although I had been living in Birmingham for four years and all my social life was there, if I returned to the house I would be at home all day by myself and tempted into doing too much. It would be unfair to rely on Cheryl and Madeleine to look after me when they came back from work during the first few weeks. So back to Blackburn it was.

Tip #46: Reduce the Shock of Discharge

Do not underestimate just how weak you are when you are discharged from hospital having had major surgery; you are so feeble it is unbelievable. In hospital you are being looked after by a small army of nurses and other staff so do not assume you can go from that to immediately looking after yourself.

Even just the two-hour car journey to Blackburn was traumatic; every minor bump on the highway seemed likely to rip open my stitches and spill my guts all over the walnut dashboard and velour trim of my parent's car. Once back at Bradley Towers though, I was able to recover by restricting my travelling to between the sofa, bathroom and spare bedroom that was my sleeping quarters for the next few weeks.

One thing that surprised me during the first two weeks' recuperation was that, despite my food intake gradually increasing towards more normal levels, my weight wasn't going up; in fact, it went down slightly. Having the good fortune to have a highly qualified nurse on hand, I learned that this was a usual occurrence, it being a sign of the intensive effort being undertaken by my body behind the scenes to repair itself.

Despite the obvious good care I was receiving at home, it was not long before I felt the urge to return to Birmingham. I had begun to think more and more about the career implications of my having Crohn's disease, and felt that the sooner I shared these thoughts with someone in Cadbury, the more likely I would be able to achieve a desirable outcome in terms of the job I would go back to. But before I addressed that issue, there was another, more pressing reason to return.

During the last few days of my incarceration on Ward 8, I had become smitten by one of the staff nurses and, on my arrival at my parents', had written her a letter suggesting a date. And, what's more, she had replied in the affirmative. So, against the advice of my mother, I packed my bags after about a four-week stay in the North and made the trip back to the house in Birmingham.

I have to report that the date was a dud, though not that the staff nurse was; in fact she was even more of a stunner out of uniform than in. (I should perhaps elaborate that "out of uniform" refers to her going-out clothes.) On the date itself, which was pleasant enough, it became increasingly apparent to me that this had been a bad idea. The cumulative trauma of my entire stay in Ward 8, coupled with her being a part of the plot, meant that I found myself talking far too much about it, which can't have been a lot of fun for her. We departed on friendly terms, but neither of us felt compelled to pick up the phone after that.

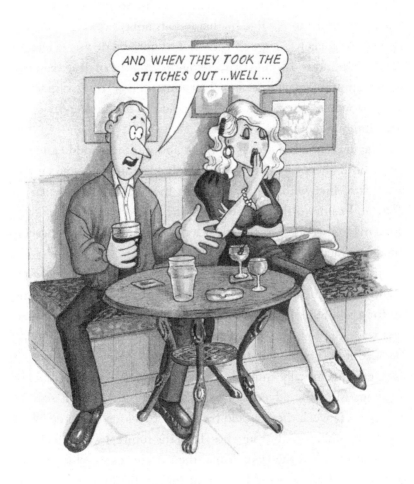

Chat-up lines from Hell

This evening out was to have a profound impact on me and on how much I would share with people, but more of that later.

The day after the date, I focused myself on my other key priority: that of planning the future direction of my career. My thinking began as follows: The hardest thing to come to terms with when dealing with Crohn's would be that it does not go away. Hence, my life was most likely going to be a series of ups and downs where, in the down periods, I would be juggling the options of drug regimes, surgery, putting up with feeling ill, or sometimes all three simultaneously. It would clearly be a mistake to add to this burden by over-stretching myself in the workplace.

Having had a few weeks to think about things, and bearing in mind both the prognosis on the probable future course of my health together with the advice from my anonymous advisor in Ward 8, I came to the conclusion that I would be foolish to continue my immediate career path as a brand manager in the marketing department.

Jobs that depended for their success on lots of doing – and brand management was a good example – would just be setting me up for a fall. Stress makes illnesses worse and being a brand manager was close to being one of the most stressful jobs in a company like Cadbury. You initiate things and have to follow them through to execution, usually multiple projects at once – plenty of ball-juggling. Also, the advertising agencies were in London, so that meant every week there would be one or two long days' travelling together with heavy-duty lunches. If, in the future, I was to feel as ill as I had done on the sales force, then these responsibilities and punishing schedules would just pour fuel on the fire.

When feeling ill, I would feel compelled to struggle into work if my absence would mean things grinding to a halt or going wrong. I did not want to do this as it would, I was now convinced, ultimately shorten my life. Conversely, if I took the time off when I was under the weather, I would ultimately fail in the job.

The question that was top of my mind was: given that Crohn's disease was for life and had already shown the level of disruption it could bring into the workplace, was there an alternative career path where I would be better able to shield the company from the new limitations I was now probably going to face? In other words, assuming the worst health-wise, how could I prevent my illness from making my employment a problem for the company and consequently for myself? But if not marketing, then what? I had been pondering these questions almost since the day I had left the hospital, but the direction I needed to take was increasingly clear.

Tip #47: You Need to be Able to Work When Feeling Ill

Look for a job that you can comfortably do when you are feeling well and get by in when you are feeling ill. Do not get into jobs where you are fully stretched when you are feeling well as you will surely fail when your health is poor. It is better to over-achieve in a role you are comfortable in rather than fail in a too demanding role.

The best kind of role for me was one that depended primarily on the quality of my thinking rather than the energy of my doing. No matter how bad I was feeling, and whether I was in the office or tucked up in bed, I could still think. This inevitably led me back to the area where I had started my career, which was much more of a thinking role. In the market analysis department, the key areas of added value were gleaning insights into reasons behind past sales performance that could be applied by colleagues in the marketing department to positively influence the future. I felt confident that I could definitely do well in that role whatever the state of my health. Plus, going back into an area I was familiar with would enable me to ease myself back into the workplace once my sick leave had run its course. So I called the personnel department and set up a meeting to discuss options for my return.

The bottom line was that I was prepared to take a step back in my career in the short term to have more control over its direction, no matter what the illness would throw at me. I was only 25 years old; I needed a long-term plan that would enable me to build a career for the next 35 years while avoiding having to choose between health and career.

Tip #48: Be the Tortoise, Not the Hare

With Crohn's, you have to plan much further ahead than you did in the past and than do others. I have met count-less people for whom Crohn's has effectively taken control of their future out of their hands, simply because they carried on as before they were ill and hoped for the best. Plan for the worst and treat anything better than that as a bonus. Stay in control of your destiny.

It turned out in the meeting that I got lucky. But as Jack Nicklaus used to say, the more he prepared, the luckier he got. Everyone was expecting that I would want to return to brand management, though not to the job I had been doing immediately prior to the surgery as that had since been filled. So they were a bit taken aback when I wheeled out my detailed pitch for a return to market analysis. I had even prepared an argument for why that department should have its staffing increased by one if, as seemed likely due to it being a small set-up, there were no vacancies.

My stroke of luck was that there was going to be a vacancy coming up in a few weeks' time. Even better, the vacancy was not for my original role as a market analyst but for the head of the section, so I would not be taking a step down at all. Now that they knew my intentions, they could put on hold their recruitment plan to fill the slot and await my return. This was excellent news for both me and the company. The job still met my criteria for being one that could stand me taking sick days when needed, in fact, probably even more so as I would be supported by a team of market analysts. For the company, it solved an immediate problem as they had no candidates lined up for the role. I was even going to get a pay rise.

We agreed on a starting date of early September, subject to my continued good progress, which meant that I would have been off work for a total of 16 weeks. Having got the job sorted out, I could now focus on ensuring as good a recovery period as possible given that I was not going to be rushing myself back in fear of losing my job. Although the days were long between Madeleine and Cheryl leaving for work and returning home, at least it was summer, so I spent a couple of hours a day sunbathing whenever the weather was nice and, when not, became addicted to daytime television – the Crohn's sufferer's best friend.

The summer also saw a gradual cranking up of my social life. A frequent visitor to my bedside in Ward 8 had been a female colleague of Cheryl's who popped by whenever her work took her to my part of the hospital. I was more than surprised to see her as, about 18 months previously, we had met at a party and had dated until I had, I am ashamed to admit, dumped her when momentarily tempted by what seemed to be, incorrectly as it turned out, a better offer. Anyway, she took the high road and was gracious enough to put my proven unreliability to one side in coming to see me during my hour of need.

As I began to feel much better during the summer, I thought I would see if she fancied carrying on where we had left off, which she did. But things didn't seem right. Firstly, chastened by my date with the nurse, I now felt very uncomfortable mentioning anything to do with Crohn's disease or the operation, but, since these topics had dominated my waking thoughts for the past several months, keeping quiet about it seemed to inhibit my socializing skills, such as they were. So, after a few nights out together, I once again called a halt, making me, I would imagine, her least impressive boyfriend ever.

After that, I lost interest in the dating game and restricted my social life to the close group of friends and family with whom I felt very comfortable. Interestingly, I was not conscious of this shift at the time; it was only pointed out to me by Madeleine during the writing of this book. It probably subconsciously flowed from the fact that I was by then rarely opening up on the subject of my health, and, on the few occasions I did so with my friends, making light of it. For example, I was quite keen to show around Cheryl's pictures of my ground-breaking surgical procedure, announcing them with the rather weak joke that they demonstrated that at least I had some guts.

But I found that talking about my Crohn's disease didn't help me feel any better; in fact it made me uncomfortable. Also, I did not want to be labeled a medical bore. I have met many medical bores in hospital clinics and I have no time for them. I have also found over the years that, while just about everyone is very quick to ask how I'm feeling at the moment, very few outside your closest friends actually want to know any details if the answer is anything other than, "Fine, thanks." You can see them glaze over almost immediately if you launch into a description of your latest drug regime and its side-effects.

Tip #49: Think About What You Share

How much you choose to share with people, either close friends or prospective new ones, is obviously a matter of personal preference. But I would strongly advise that you base your decision not just on what you want to do, but on the receptiveness and interest level of your audience. Don't make your illness into a problem for others.

During the balmy days of August, I was beginning to think about all the wonderful initiatives I would unleash on my return to the workplace. I made a return visit to see Dr. Ray who informed me that my condition seemed excellent. Of course, this was the kiss of death, or to be more accurate, the embrace of relapse. Almost as soon as I had returned home from seeing him, there was evidence that my illness was once again on the prowl. What had been for me in the glory days of the summer an almost unheard-of once only daily toilet habit become twice and then more. Equally, a rare bloodspot became a regular event along with an occasionally quite bloodstained tissue.

Although I had steeled myself to the notion that my Crohn's was for life and that symptoms would someday return, I found it impossible to contemplate that it might have returned before I had even gone back to work. What happened to the five years promised me by the surgeon? Perhaps he had neglected to mention that four years and nine months of that might entail enduring more of the same symptoms which I had thought the surgery would banish. However, despite my unwillingness to contemplate an almost immediate return of symptoms, I had to accept what was going on, so I very reluctantly picked up the phone and booked myself in to see Doctor Ray.

Return to Jail

"I'm not feeling very well, I need a doctor immediately. Ring the nearest golf course."

> **– Groucho Marx**

AS I WAS now just a regular patient, I didn't have the benefit of a senior registrar from the surgical team to browbeat Dr. Ray into seeing me personally and immediately, so I had been put onto the list for the inflammatory bowel patients' clinic that took place every Thursday afternoon. Once I had checked in with the receptionist, I was able to take a seat in the corridor and observe how the system worked.

It was immediately apparent that this was a big production number. There were several patients waiting alongside me with more arriving every few minutes. On an irregular but frequent basis, a doctor would pop his or her head into the corridor and summon a patient. I soon ascertained that there were three doctors apart from Dr. Ray involved in what was a very high throughput clinic. This was clearly another case where a collection of medical problems had been transformed into a logistical problem, being addressed by multiple doctors with extremely short consultations. I clearly wasn't going to get much one-on-one time with whoever called out my name.

The means by which patients were allocated doctors was as low tech as it comes. Once checked in, my notes folder was placed underneath an existing pile of other patients' folders, and every time a doctor sent a patient off to the next stage of the production line – a blood test – they would take the folder on the top of the pile and return to their lair, study it for a couple of minutes at most, then summon the patient in. Complete chance as to who I would get, and unless they were Olympic speed-readers, they would know only the bare minimum about my case when I walked in for my speed-consult.

The various doctors were also clearly of very different ages and, one would assume, expertise. This set me thinking that the more cases a doctor had seen, the more likely they would be to recognize obscure complications. It wasn't that I had anything against youth, it was simply a question of experience. Equally, I had nothing against a doctor's country of origin, but again it came down to experience. The incidence of Crohn's disease varies dramatically across the globe. If a young doctor was trained in a country where Crohn's is very rare, e.g. Singapore, where an internet search informs me that only 8,000 out of four million inhabitants are stricken, then they probably hadn't seen many cases like mine.

Tip #50: Try to Influence Which Doctor You See

It's always a good idea to figure out the logistics of whatever clinic you have to attend. It may be as simple as asking the receptionist when you check in if you can see a certain doctor that day. She may, of course, tell you to get stuffed, but nothing ventured, nothing gained. Not a problem in the U.S., of course, where one gets to see the doctor of one's choice.

Having not yet sussed out for myself that I could have been doing more to get to see the right doctor, I stayed in the random selection process and drew the short straw when summonsed by a very youthful-looking doctor who indeed turned out to be the student there to study Crohn's disease at the feet of the master.

"So", he commenced after we both sat down, "How have you been?"

I had already figured out while waiting and observing that, if I wanted to get a result from this visit, I had to adjust my tactics to suit the situation, i.e. an extremely limited amount of time and a doctor who it was best to assume knew nothing whatsoever about my case. Doctors see dozens of patients in what can seem a bewildering flurry of similar but subtly different cases when they don't have the time to spend 30 minutes poring over each set of notes.

If I was to ramble on and not really get to the point of what had changed and why I was there, then I couldn't really blame him if he defaulted to my case being "typical" and then give me stock responses and placebo treatments. So I had already prepared in my head a summarized version of events, leading into an update on my current symptoms and finishing off with a question along the lines of, "Is this normal for just three months after surgery?"

Tip #51: Prepare for Every Medical Consultation

It is a good idea to be thoroughly prepared for every medical consultation, no matter who you think you are seeing and for how long. It comes down to you taking ownership for what happens in the consultation. This is a critical component of becoming a successful Crohn's patient.

By summarizing my case history, giving a clear and brief update on the new news and then making it clear what was on my mind, I was, in effect, doing most of this doctor's job for him. You may feel that he's getting paid a lot of money to be able to do that for himself, but, in the situation of a busy clinic, you have to help them to help you.

I was correct in surmising that the return of some of my symptoms was not the normal course of events after such surgery. He explained to me that the strictureplasty technique was primarily to resolve the problems associated with blockage. Although a big chunk of badly inflamed bowel had also been removed, there could well have been some active inflammation in the strictures themselves that would not have been resolved by the surgery as strictureplasties do not remove any tissue. So, although my symptoms of blockage had indeed disappeared, if the inflammation still in there had flared up again, then that would account for there being some of my old symptoms. He wasn't bad for a student.

That being the case, the way forward was to consider the various drug treatments that at the time constituted the arsenal against inflammation, together with something to slow my bowels down and sort out the, by now, ever-present mild-to-moderate diarrhea. The fail-safe in the clinic procedure to cover for the fact that not all the doctors were equally knowledgeable was that any change in medication, which included the introduction of medication, had to be run past Dr. Ray. So the young medic toddled off for a quick meet and returned a couple of minutes later with the plan.

It transpired that, in some cases, a quick course of tablets that dampened down inflammation could lead not just to a temporary respite from symptoms, but result in the induction of a period of remission, settling down the inflammation such that it would stay subdued without the need for ongoing medication. And there was a range of drugs that apparently had some kind of track record of achieving this effect. True to the edict contained in the Hippocratic Oath that the first rule of doctoring is to do no harm, or as little harm as possible, the plan was to start with the most innocuous drug and see what happened. The drug in question was called Salazopirin, which would also be joined by another drug that I would take every day to control my loose bowel, that being one called Codeine Phosphate. So here commenced what would be a feature of my life from that point onwards: prescription drugs.

It becomes obvious very quickly when you are prescribed a drug therapy that the drug in question can do various things to you other than meeting its stated purpose. As we all know from the sheets of warnings that now accompany any prescription, these come under the heading of "side effects". This, in my view, is a term that must have been cooked up by the marketing and PR gurus at the drug companies, as I find it highly misleading. We are encouraged to believe that the technical geniuses have formulated the drug to primarily perform the task in hand but, due to the limitations of science, it may, just may, on very rare occasions, do something else to you as well.

This myth was shattered for me within an hour of being given a prescription for my two drugs as I once again detoured into Birmingham Central Library to read up on them. Salazopirin seemed to be innocuous enough, it being listed as an anti-inflammatory, but Codeine Phosphate immediately gave the game away. Much to my surprise, the stated purpose of this drug was firstly as pain relief followed by a secondary role as a cough suppressant. Eh? Delving into the small print of side effects, I found, along with double-vision, dizziness, drowsiness, dry mouth, headache, loss of appetite (great!), nausea (double great!) and unusual tiredness or weakness (oh, come on, is this a joke???) – constipation. I was being prescribed this drug for one of its supposed side effects.

Of course, in this day and age of computer technology and cut 'n' paste, the drug companies can plug such a breach in their communication strategy by simply elevating to the top of the list the effect that the patient requires the drug for and relegate the previous front-runner back into the following pack of "side effects." But in those days, it had to be printed once and for all in black and white. So someone had, no doubt, played the percentages game and listed the effects in proportion to the ailments for which the drug was, on average, prescribed.

I also learned that Codeine Phosphate was a narcotic and hence subject to a much longer list of side effects that did not constitute possible treatments for anything, such as: depression, pounding heartbeat, feelings of unreality, hallucinations, increased sweating, irregular breathing, flushed face, ringing in the ears, wheezing, swelling of the face, trembling, pinpoint eye pupils and, for good measure, seizures. These, when added together, sounded like how Keith Richards must feel all the time. No wonder he looks like he does.

There are no free rides with medication; every drug floods through your veins and washes over every cell in your body. You just have to hope that the drug effects that alleviate your symptoms outweigh the other effects that make you feel worse. Also, do not be surprised if the drug has no beneficial effect whatsoever. The New York Times reported on December 30, 2008 that, "most drugs, whatever the disease, work for only about half the people who take them."

Tip #52: Balance Beneficial Effects Against Side Effects

If you feel you are on the wrong end of the side-effect trade-off, or feel that you are one of the 50% for whom the drug is useless anyway, do not hesitate to go back and demand a change in medication. There are usually several different drugs which purport to improve a certain set of symptoms; keep on changing until you find the one that causes you least harm relative to the improvement it gives.

I can report that my two drugs matched the New York Times average. The Codeine Phosphate did indeed help slow down my bowels, with the added benefits of me never having a headache and never having a cough. However, the Salazopirin, after a promising start, proved to be useless. So, with the addition of abdominal pain to my list of symptoms, back I went to the clinic a couple of months later and thought I had hit the jackpot when Dr. Ray himself was the one who picked my notes up from the pile and summoned me into his inner sanctum.

The location of my pain, on the right-hand side of my abdomen, was clearly mystifying to him so, much to my horror, he announced that another Barium enema was required to check what was going on in my colon. Once again, I did the starvation, purgative, butt-clenching routine and was back in his office a couple of weeks later for the post-match summary, which confirmed that things looked a bit questionable in the colon. This came as a shock to me as the surgery had not involved my colon at all and I knew from my library researches that this could be bad news, bringing images of colostomy bags floating into my mind. His response to this news was, thankfully, less dramatic, involving only the doubling of my dosage of Salazopirin and a booking to come back and see him in a month's time.

So I dutifully returned four weeks later and avoided the trainees as Dr. Ray made a point of taking my notes from the waiting pile, even though I was still far from the top. Good news that I was seeing the top banana; bad news that I was on his watch list. The consultation was uneventful, the plan being to give this useless drug another four weeks and, if things were no better, he planned to add another drug to the cocktail, Metronidazole. By now I was not even surprised when my research dug up the news that this new drug was an antibiotic used to treat, amongst other things, vaginal thrush. The side effects were not particularly frightening, an ever-present metallic taste being the only one I suffered, but the really bad news was that alcohol had to be avoided at all costs. Boooo!

Four weeks later I was back again feeling a bit brighter, but it was at this consultation that things began to go wrong, something I was unaware of until many years later when I took advantage of Britain's Freedom of Information Act to get a copy of my medical notes. The letter following this consultation from Dr. Ray to my family doctor began innocently enough, "He has been rather better in the last two weeks." But then came the zinger, "He seems to have had post-operative depression, and I have strongly reassured him that the future is brighter." Wrong on both counts.

Words cannot express how angry I felt when I eventually read this, and my mother's response made mine seem like a mild frustration. We were, and still are, outraged. Everyone who knows me well would confirm that I am a positive person; I do not suffer from depression. How was it that a man who barely knew me could have jumped to such an erroneous conclusion? Surely the logical interpretation of my glum face was that of extreme disappointment that the symptoms had returned while I was still recuperating from the surgery. I would have thought this would not be difficult to comprehend, but no, in the eyes of the medical profession apparently I was depressed and hence imagining symptoms.

It only became apparent to me years down the line that his judgment on this issue was being led by the fact that the symptoms I was reporting didn't match up to what the regular blood tests were telling him, specifically, what my Erythrocyte Sedimentation Rate was telling him. In this test, the tube of drawn blood is left to stand upright. Red blood cells, known as erythrocytes in the phlebotomy business, gradually fall to the bottom of the tube to form a sludge leaving the clear plasma at the top – a kind of reverse pint of

Guinness effect. The rate at which they collect at the bottom is measured and compared to norms. If they fall more quickly than average, that is usually because they are covered by a sticky protein that, as a rule, is pumped into the bloodstream at the site of any inflammation.

You no doubt have already spotted the problem here: "Norms", "average", "usually", "as a rule". In other words, this test was not infallible. But doctors, who think all animals that create hoof-beats are horses, also think that a test which holds true most of the time is good enough all of the time. Doctors pay a lot more attention to the tests than they do to the patient because tests are scientific whereas patients are most definitely not. If there is a mismatch between the test and the patient's complaining, then, more often than not, the assumption will be that is because the patient is most likely a wildly exaggerating manic depressive.

Tip #53: When Symptoms Don't Match Test Results, Stand Firm

With a lifetime condition such as Crohn's, where the course of the illness varies by patient and we have hundreds of medical tests, this will happen to you one day. The doctor will not believe what you are saying because some test is indicating otherwise. If you think that is happening, change your doctor, because once they label you as a depressive, then that will color every judgment they make from that point on.

This misperception on his part would be a detriment to my treatment for the next ten years. It is now obvious to me that the signs were there that I was rapidly heading for his "too difficult" pile.

This is where your symptoms resist the efforts of the doctors to get them under control which with Crohn's is a bad place to be. When you stubbornly refuse to get better, doctors do not go into Sherlock Holmes mode and see this as a three-pipe-problem to test their skills and knowledge. More often, they refuse to accept that their years of training are failing to get the job done and conclude that there must be another explanation, i.e. you are not as ill as you are saying. But I knew nothing of this at the time. I had appreciated his fatherly chat and had believed his platitudes that the corner was about to be turned.

So, when three months later in April 1984 I was back again, grumbling about my symptoms, the subsequent letter to the family doctor focused on the fact that my blood count, profile and ESR were all normal and that he had reassured me and booked me in for two weeks' time. Two weeks' time – same again. One month's time – ditto. In July, it seems he had a tiny sliver of doubt in the tests and gave me a prescription for the strong stuff, which, for Crohn's patients, is steroids. Not anabolic steroids – the body-builders' drug of choice – but Prednisolone.

Again, another trip to the library filled me in on the details, which were far too extensive for me to fully repeat here. The key points were that this was actually an artificial version of a substance produced naturally in the body by the adrenal gland and had a list of frightening effects as long as your arm. However, it was the most potent weapon in the anti-inflammatory armory so would have the best chance of settling me down.

The usual regime was a short time spent on a high dose to shock any inflammation into submission, followed by a gradual reduction in dosage to wean you off it. This weaning is necessary because taking the drug switches off your body's ability to manufacture nature's own version. If you stop taking the drug suddenly, your body can't crank up production quickly enough which leaves you vulnerable to all sorts of horrible ways of dying as you do actually need this stuff in your system all the time. Even though it mimicked a natural substance, the amount prescribed in the short, sharp shock phase was several times the body's natural levels so there was no chance of me not noticing I was taking it.

I can best describe it as nature's rocket fuel; I felt like a character from Marvel Comics as my appetite and energy levels went through the roof. I only needed about four hours' sleep a night and seemed to spend the other twenty hours eating – a sort of cross between Popeye and Fatty Arbuckle. Prior to me taking this hi-octane drug, my appetite, which had briefly rallied following the surgery, had slumped back to its pre-operative status of me miserably pushing food around my plate. However, within a week of starting the steroids, I was eating a large breakfast to start the day; a plate-full of meat and vegetables in the Cadbury canteen for lunch; a large evening meal and a plate of sandwiches halfway during the night; and I was still permanently hungry! While I hadn't been able to look at food before my operation, I now couldn't stop looking for it.

The weight piled on. From being a pathetic 126-pound weakling straight out of the "Before" part of a Charles Atlas ad, I soon had the bathroom scales begging for mercy as I topped 140 pounds, then 155 and was heading towards 170 with no sign of slowing down. My entire wardrobe was now functionally useless, forcing me to go on a Paris Hilton-esque shopping spree. After an entire adult lifetime spent in the "Small" category, I was now exploring not just the "Mediums" but the occasional "Large". I loved it!

The slowdown came as I gradually reduced the dosage as per my instructions, but this, much to my dismay, also coincided with the very unwelcome gradual return of my symptoms. I visited Dr.

Ray's clinic every month for several months in a row as we wrestled with the dilemma that I was unable to get off the steroids without feeling ill again. Each time the dosage was bumped up I felt marvelous only for me to gradually decline as the dosage diminished. The problem with this state of affairs was that higher dosages of steroids come with a host of quite dramatic effects along with the appetite and the energy.

Fluid retention had swelled my face up into the typical steroid "moon-face" visage such that I really didn't recognize myself. This effect struck me most forcefully when I was having my hair cut and would be staring at a complete stranger in the mirror for half an hour at a time. There was also terrible acne on my back, so much so that I was unwilling to take off my t-shirt even when swimming. I was also, for the first time in my life, subject to quite extreme mood swings. I'm normally a Steady-Eddie kind of guy so it came as a complete shock to find myself getting extremely uptight at work over what would normally be barely noticeable irritations. Eventually, it was decided that I should stay on a low dose, only slightly higher than the body's own natural supply, as this seemed the best compromise between illness and adverse effects. But it was not all downside.

As I was feeling a lot better on the steroids, I had begun ratcheting up my social life again, although nothing serious in terms of relationships had developed as I was still reticent to fully share with others. However, this would all be swept away by the culmination of my return to socializing which came when I was struck by the proverbial thunderbolt. I had been cajoled by one of the secretaries in the marketing department to buy two tickets to her netball club dance, to which I had gone along with a friend, Rob, who was by now my main drinking partner. Rob had a bit of a thing for another of the secretaries so he was keen to come along. When he saw her on the dance floor with her best friend, he forced me into accompanying him in asking them if they minded us joining them.

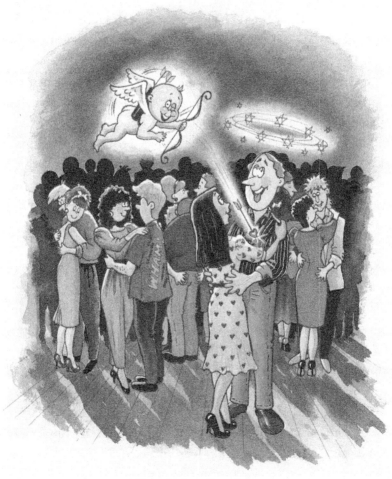

Save the last dance for me

The friend, Audrey, was another secretary in the marketing department and someone I had met on my first day there. By this time I had been at Cadbury nearly five years and we knew each other well.

Although we had indulged in a slow dance at a previous Christmas party, our relationship had been platonic. But this time, as we danced away, I was hit squarely in the heart by cupid's arrow. I got the full works: stars flashed in my eyes, my heart raced, I could hardly breathe. How could I have been so blind? Here was this girl, beautiful in both looks and spirit, who had been under my nose for years. The clincher was when, in between dances, she confessed that she had initially had a crush on me when I had first joined the company. I shied away from making my move there and then, but began plotting my attack immediately I got back into the office.

My opportunity came a week later when a colleague in the market research department invited us both "plus partner" to his wedding evening reception. Since neither I nor Audrey was currently plus partner, I suggested that we go together. It turned out that she had been as smitten as me at the netball disco, so my elaborately prepared chat-up lines were largely left unused. Within two weeks, I knew this was the person I wanted to spend the rest of my life with.

I then began to plot where and when to propose to her. Common sense told me that two weeks was a bit Britney Spears in terms of a courtship, so I managed to restrain myself for another two months, popping the question on her birthday during a weekend away in south Wales, staying at the very hotel in Swansea where I had been on the sales force. My miserable memories of having stayed there for months on end while I was so ill were wiped away in an instant when Audrey said, "Yes". In fact, she said, "Yes, yes, yes, yes, yes YES!!!," giving me the distinct impression that I had, in her opinion, been somewhat slow in popping the question.

There is no doubt in my mind that, if I hadn't been on the steroids, I wouldn't have gone to the dance, wouldn't have asked Audrey out, wouldn't have fallen in love, wouldn't have popped the question and wouldn't have spent the next 25 years with the most wonderful person on earth.

Tip #54: Look For the Unexpected Benefits

Like anything in life, there is always an upside, and that applies to having Crohn's. Illness takes your life in a different direction, leading you to new crossroads and new opportunities. You must view these new choices, not in the light of what they would have been if you hadn't have been ill, but what they offer as new potential life-paths.

Given that Audrey had won my heart so completely, I had dropped my reticence in not talking about my health and had been very open with her from the start as to what had happened in the past and what the future might hold. Soon after our engagement, I crystallized this approach in a conversation with Audrey along the lines of, "Do you know what you are letting yourself in for with my health?" At this point, I shall pass the keyboard to her and ask her to explain how she felt on the subject.

"I suspect that no matter how graphic or detailed John could have been about explaining the complexities of what our married life together with the omnipresent Crohn's disease might hold, my reply to his marriage proposal would not have been anything other than "yes, yes, yes" (which were, indeed, my exact words), because, by then, I was well and truly in love with him. In fact, just for the record, I believe I was in love with him from the very first moment we met way back in 1979; it just took him a little longer to figure it out!

"I had seen how poorly John looked when he returned to the department from the sales force, and had also visited him in hospital after his first operation along with other work colleagues, so I already had a vague idea of what this disease was capable of. That said, nothing can prepare you for the heartbreak when witnessing what John has had and continues to endure at the hands of this disease.

"I could already see, even back then, John's determination not to allow his illness, whilst always being part of our lives, to dominate. It can sometimes be somewhat challenging to remain strong whilst seeing someone you love to their very core in such pain and distress but it definitely brings home the commitment we made to one another on our wedding day 'for better, for worse'. Right from the start of our relationship, we particularly tried to focus on the 'better' with the guarantee that 'worse' almost certainly waited in the wings."

Thank you, Audrey. We married on May 18, 1985, and our wedding pictures pay testament to the effects of the steroids that I was still taking: the fat guy next to her looks nothing like me.

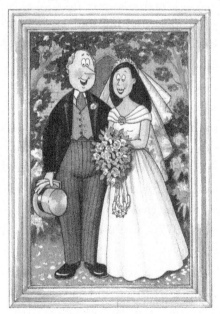

The More Things Change...

"Formerly, when religion was strong and science weak, men mistook magic for medicine; now, when science is strong and religion weak, men mistake medicine for magic."
— Thomas Szasz, Hungarian psychiatrist, 1920 -

WITHIN A MONTH of getting married, the steroids also had a beneficial effect on my career, when I successfully applied for a job back in the marketing department. Why, you may ask, did I renege on my very sensible plan to steer clear of a stressful career in marketing? The answer is that, while taking the steroids, I not only felt much better and capable of stepping up to a more taxing role, but I now believe that they were making me more effective and assertive in the workplace, to the point where I had become somewhat bored in my current back-room job. But I did not completely ignore my own advice; the job I went for was one which I felt was uniquely suited to the limitations that my health would inflict if and when I eventually was taken off steroids.

My thinking had evolved since immediately after the operation. It was still the case that I felt I should avoid jobs that demanded long hours and plenty of travel, but I had also realized through my success in my current role that a key component was it being the kind of role where, if I felt unwell, I did not feel intense pressure to drag myself into work the next day. The role I applied for was the only one in the marketing arena that fulfilled both criteria.

The job in question was responsible for Cadbury's ranges of Easter and Christmas products. The job was mainly based in Birmingham and involved very rare travel to London, but the clincher for me was that, like with most seasonal categories such as firecrackers and gardening implements, there were very long timescales involved. The product ranges were sold to customers 10 months ahead of time and then production was geared to meet the orders that came in. That meant that the development work that formed the role's key responsibility took place in the 12 months prior to that. In effect, the job was working two years ahead of when the products would actually be in the shops. My thinking was that, if I didn't feel well, then being off sick tomorrow would most likely not have a catastrophic impact on sales that would not happen for another 18 months. There would always be time to catch back up again.

It was at this point I worked out that living with Crohn's is like navigating Macy's via the escalators where the goal is to get to the top floor. When feeling well, it is time to get on the next set of escalators and go up to the next floor. When feeling ill, one should spend time on the floor, content to browse through the goods for a while. If you try to just keep going up escalators, whether feeling well or ill, you will at some stage fall off.

My job in marketing services had been spending time on one of the floors; my move back into marketing and also proposing to Audrey had been progressing up to the next level while I was feeling well enough to do so. If I had stayed in my comfortable marketing services role and remained a social hermit, I would have missed the opportunity to get further towards fulfilling my work potential and my life's happiness without jeopardizing my long-term health.

Tip #55: Slow, Slow, Quick-Quick, Slow

The trick is to be ambitious when you are feeling well and cautious when you are not. Do not miss out on sensible opportunities because you got into the habit of not pushing yourself. Equally, do not make things worse by always pushing yourself, even when you feel terrible.

I am glad I pushed myself when I did, because if I had left it a couple of years, I would have missed out on the escalator. But I don't think either of us was expecting that the illness would play such a big part in our early married life.

In preparing to get into bed one evening, as I sat on the edge of the bed I felt a slight, but still sharp, shooting pain deep in the nether regions. I was in little doubt that this was a reoccurrence of the dreaded perianal abscess. I knew that steroids weakened the body's immune system and thus assumed that the abscess had been lingering in there and was now taking its unexpected opportunity to put in a repeat appearance.

As the next day was a Thursday, I was able to book myself into that day's Ward 8 clinic to seek immediate attention before it worsened into the crippling event I had endured just prior to my operation. I wasn't really bothered which doctor saw me as surely an abscess would have been something even the laziest dullard to have ever graduated from medical school would have been able to recognize. I don't recall which doctor I saw, probably because for most of our encounter he was out of my field of vision, staring at and then digitally probing my rear end. Not much fun for either of us.

Anyway, I got the result I wanted, which was an invitation, amazingly, to check into Ward 8 the next day and have the surgeons deal with the matter before it followed the same, predictable course and completely crippled me. I think in hindsight that the unexpected speed of response in getting me booked in was due to the not insignificant risk of having such a rampant infection in my body while my immune system was taking a steroid-induced vacation.

The procedure was event-free as I stayed asleep during the operation and woke up after, and not before, the curare had worn off. This being classed as a minor procedure, I only ever saw the mid-ranking member of the surgical team who had been entrusted with the comparatively simple task. However, he had used a bit of imagination and creativity during the procedure, having decided that two occurrences of an abscess in the same area represented a trend and hence this was a problem that could well keep rearing its ugly head (or heading into my ugly rear).

The permanent solution was that he had not merely cleaned out the infection but had opened up the path to the infection site with the follow-up plan to allow the abscess site to heal from the inside out. This would be accomplished by packing the wound with a dressing to allow drainage and healing. I think I was only in the ward for an overnight stop before being sent on my way with the welcome news that I would need to have a good couple of weeks off work to heal.

During this time, I would have to either not sit down or re-employ my trusty rubber-ring. I would also be visited every couple of days by a home nurse who would change the wound dressing, gradually decreasing its bulk as the abscess cavity filled itself in by rebuilding layers of flesh. I had a mental image of a home nurse being a sort of steely-eyed, gray-haired battleaxe, a kind of General Patton with a stethoscope, whereas the one who was assigned my case was more Nurse Chapel from Star Trek. She was also clearly operating under a similar expectation that her patient would be a grey-haired, grumpy oldster as she seemed taken aback when I opened the door and confirmed that I was indeed her next patient.

To our mutual discomfort, I led this young lady to the bedroom and, while she wandered off to wash her hands, I dropped the pants and assumed the position. There could be no pretence at modesty given the task she had to complete, the only benefit being that I didn't have to look her in the eye while she fiddled around between my splayed legs due to me being face down biting the pillow. I am often asked how I deal with these moments. Normally I would use humor but I have found that weak jokes only add to the tension as they just signal how uncomfortable you really are. Plus, nurses have already heard many times every joke you can think of involving butts, so a dignified silence is my preferred approach.

It is now obvious to me that this was not a reawakening of the first abscess brought back to life by the steroids, but was a separate event brought about by the return of my Crohn's disease. The steroids were doing a marvelous job of making me feel well, which I mistakenly interpreted as that they were working and my Crohn's disease had been stopped in its tracks.

Tip #56: Never Assume That Your Medicine is Actually Working

While you don't want to obsessively worry over every little thing that happens to you, it's a good discipline to at least consider the possibility that your treatment might not be working. Don't always accept the easiest, most optimistic explanation, which in this case was along the lines of, "It's probably the remnants of the last abscess." At least ask, "Just supposing it is a new manifestation of my illness, would we be doing anything different at this stage? Is there anything I should be looking out for?"

Once healed, my next visit to Dr. Ray saw a different outcome to the usual wait-and-see approach. The abscess added to his concerns that all was not well in my large bowel, so another barium enema was ordered. His note to the family doctor backtracked on previous editions by admitting that perhaps it was not all in my head and that further surgical treatment might be required to restore me to good health. However, the results of the enema were inconclusive so we went back to waiting and seeing.

The next medical event should have been the clincher that surgery was inevitable, but I failed to inform the medics at the time as I misinterpreted what was going on. Audrey and I had gone down to London for the weekend having been invited to a party at Madeleine's, who by this point had left Cadbury's, the shared house and Birmingham to work for Sainsbury's supermarket chain (head office rather than the checkout). I awoke the morning after the party with an overwhelmingly intense nausea coupled with occasional crippling stomach spasms. I did not even consider that this might be a Crohn's-related intestinal blockage as the symptoms were very different to the blockages I had endured in the past and while selling chocolate in deepest west Wales. I was a lot more bothered by the nausea than the pain, and this had never been a feature of what I considered the blockage set of symptoms.

I tried to eat a little breakfast cereal but that only made me feel worse. Then we tried going out for some fresh air only for me to end up dry-retching in the middle of Safeway's parking lot (and not just at their prices). When we returned to our lodgings, I tried to induce further vomiting by the trusty method of drinking salt water, but it merely came back up again without resolving the worsening symptoms. Our thinking was that this must just be an exceptionally bad reaction to something I had eaten the night before.

Since nothing seemed to be helping, we decided that, as I would feel just as ill wherever I was, Audrey would drive us both back home to Birmingham. By this point I was bordering on the semi-delirious and, as we hit the road, was drifting in and out of a pain-racked sleep. However, I came to with a jolt when my body's early-warning system flagged up to me that I was going to vomit. But unfortunately the warning was not early enough. Before I had time to register where I was, a stream of vomit blasted the dashboard as though from a fire hose, bouncing up onto the windscreen and then back over me. It made the scene in The Exorcist look like a mild case of acid reflux.

When I had last remembered being awake, Audrey, who was not comfortable driving my rather flashy and speedy car, had been crawling along in the inside lane at little old lady speed, clutching the steering wheel as though her life depended on it. During the period I had been out of it, she had clearly adapted to the speedster and, when I woke up to redecorate the car interior, she was hammering along in the outside lane, steering with one hand while leaning on the horn and flashing the headlights at anyone foolish enough to not get out of her way.

The explosion to her left-hand side amazingly did not faze her and she immediately began forcefully weaving her way through the lanes of traffic to head towards the median strip. However, not quite fast enough. I felt another digestive tsunami coming up fast so I opened the door and leaned out, leaving a trail of vomit a good hundred yards long through the middle and inner lanes as she tacked through the traffic and drew to a halt.

As I stared wretchedly at the asphalt, I couldn't help noticing that this was not the vomit I recollected from days of my youth following drinking binges in the fleshpots of Blackburn. Where were the diced carrots? In fact, there were no bits whatsoever; and it wasn't vomit-colored but a deep brown. The mystery deepened when one final heave brought up another puddle into which plopped a perfectly formed button mushroom. This one little mushroom was the only evidence of any solid matter. And then I felt better. Instantly.

I had no explanation for this sequence of events. I had gone from feeling worse than I ever imagined possible to feeling quite normal in the space of less than a minute. Well, as normal as one can do when both oneself and one's prized car were covered in a strange and quite horrible-smelling vomit. The journey then continued uneventfully, with all the windows open, Audrey having the good sense to head for her parents house where I could recuperate from the ordeal while her father was handed the gruesome task of cleaning up the car.

I only realized much later that the not-very-well-chewed mushroom had got stuck at a stricture like a cork in a wine bottle. Mushrooms are not very pliable and also do not break down easily in the digestive juices, so my system had given up trying to push it through the stricture and then abandoned the body's Plan B of waiting for it to dissolve. Fortunately, the body has a back-up third alternative, this being known as projectile vomiting, for good reason, as it reverses the flow of the digestive system and sends the entire contents of your digestive system from your socks upwards back up with enough force to stucco a house from the other side of the street. The much darker color of the vomit was due to it not just being the hardly digested stomach contents, but the much more digested contents of the small intestine.

The stricture explanation only became obvious to me when I had another blockage problem a couple of months later. This time I knew exactly what it was and was even aware that it was going to happen a few hours before it did. I was eating an apple and carelessly swallowed a very large piece that almost choked me on the way down. As soon as it was past the point of no return, I feared the worst, which duly came about a few hours later. But I was spared the projectile heaving as, although the blockage pain was intense and lasted for several hours, the apple was finally eaten away by the digestive system's hydrochloric acid and eventually slipped through the stricture without having to come all the way back up again.

Tip #57: Tell the Doctor Everything, No Matter How Unrelated.

I did not mention the mushroom event the next time I visited the Ward 8 clinic as I did not think it was related to my Crohn's and assumed was probably due to some suspect seafood. Never assume anything. Even if the medic is yawning, looking at her watch and tapping her pencil on the desk, mention everything that has happened since your last visit, no matter how unrelated it might seem to you.

However, the apple event was one I could not pass off as being unrelated and duly reported it at the next clinic. The way I related the event was planned to leave no doubt in any doctor's mind that it had indeed been caused by a stricture. Now I knew the stricture was there, I didn't want to be fobbed off with a "see if it happens again" response due to me giving a woolly description. For good measure, I also threw in the Mystery of the Mushroom, which the medic did indeed confirm as a rather dramatic example of a blockage that would not unblock. He also passed on the news that, if the body's own projectile vomiting system had not cleared the blockage, then the only other solution would have been an emergency surgery. Eeeek!

The thought that I might have been operated on in some North London district hospital by an average hacker went against all my learning so far about living with Crohn's, with the emphasis on "living". The last thing I wanted was to have to undergo surgery in some Hicksville set-up where the surgeon may never have seen a stricture. Surgeons, in my experience, are not the kind of people who readily admit self-doubt and will press on and operate with a supreme confidence that might be completely unjustified.

Tip #58: Don't Become an Emergency

You have to plan ahead to avoid being operated on at the wrong time in the wrong place by the wrong surgeon. It is a statistical fact that 50% of surgeons qualified in the lower half of their cohort. Add to that the fact that there are many different procedures they will have had little to no experience of, which might include yours. You need to get operated on ideally in a university-affiliated teaching hospital by a real specialist who can do your particular procedure in his sleep, having done it hundreds of times and having seen every possible complication. Don't keep putting things off and then turn into an emergency case.

Bearing this in mind, I was more than amenable to the suggestion that a good next step would be to undergo another barium meal to ascertain just how bad this stricture was. While I was waiting for that appointment to come round, I made sure I chewed my food to a smooth paste to avoid any repetition.

The barium meal took place a couple of weeks later and, as I now considered myself an experienced at this, I concentrated more on craning my neck to see the screen showing the live X-rays of the gloop making its way through the system. As I had been paying attention on the day I was diagnosed when Dr. Ray talked me through my X-rays, I now knew what a stricture looked like, and was able to spot at least three of them on-screen during the procedure.

After I had sent the barium on its next step towards the Birmingham sewage treatment works, the radiologist, in response to my asking what he had discovered, tersely informed me that he would write up his report and send it to Dr. Ray, from whom I would hear in due course. Radiologists aren't much into giving out spontaneous diagnoses and can be counted on to play a bunt and give nothing away whatsoever. I naturally assumed that I would be summonsed to attend the Ward 8 clinic to get a personal debrief but, much to my surprise, the next thing I received was a letter from Doctor Ray. In this letter, he confirmed that the barium meal had highlighted numerous strictures but that, since I was otherwise feeling well, we would "see how things went."

I was not happy to read this. The thought that a momentary lapse in my chewing could land me in a surgical emergency worried me greatly. If this emergency situation did indeed happen, not only was I concerned about not seeing the very best Crohn's surgeon, but a completely unexpected three months off work would wreak havoc with my strategy of not letting my illness be a problem for Cadbury.

My unhappiness was added to with the fact that the only reason I was feeling well was because of the steroids, which was not a sustainable treatment anyway. Long-term steroid use carries all sorts of risks such as diabetes, weakened bones and even dementia. After discussing the situation with both Audrey and my mother, I wrote back to Dr. Ray making as strong a case as I could for a planned surgery to resolve all these new strictures, ideally in a few weeks' time so I could make arrangements at work for my area to tick over in my absence.

I don't know if doctors usually get letters from patients demanding major surgery. Probably not, so I didn't know what to expect in terms of a response. Would I be summonsed to the clinic to get a lecture on who made the medical decisions around here? Or would it merely be filed in the round mesh filing cabinet as the ravings of yet another deranged patient?

Tip #59: For Something Really Important, Send a Letter.

Do not assume that you cannot initiate communication with doctors if you have something on your mind. Bear in mind that the clinic situation is not always the best venue as you might be rushed, or even not see the doctor you want to see. A letter can be a good way of getting across your perspective as you have the time to formulate your arguments properly.

I never actually heard back from Dr. Ray and had just got to the point of assuming that the letter had been thrown away when I received a computer-generated appointment form telling me to present myself to the Royal Free Hospital Admissions Department in another couple of weeks' time for my surgery. So the letter had clearly worked. Getting, on a planned basis, the surgery that would put my mind at rest and hopefully finally resolve the stricture problem was the kind of progress I wanted to be making as opposed to "seeing how things go." Also, it was an eye-opener for me in terms of the influence I had been able to have on the course of my medical treatment.

Tip #60: Ask For What You Want

If you conduct yourself in a professional manner as a patient then you can build a level of credibility with the medics such that your point of view on treatment is taken on board. While you will most likely survive, you cannot thrive as a Crohn's patient by being completely passive with the medics.

Audrey was feeling a lot less positive than me about this turn of events. I was focused on the longer-term benefits of being in control of both my health and my career. She, on the other hand, was sick with worry about me having a major surgery that had not been without incident last time around. We had only been married for six months at this point, so it was not the start to our life together she had imagined. I made my arrangements at work confirming I would be off for fourteen weeks or so, then the day before my appointment was due, began the starvation process and packed my hospital long-stay survival kit.

The next day, a taxi duly appeared at 9am and off I went back to my second home – Ward 8. Once bedded in, as a seasoned veteran, I could spend my time more focused on what was going on around me rather than worrying about what was going to happen to me. The first thing I noticed was that there had been a changing of the guard in the ward staffing. Sister Grey had gone and had been replaced by one of the staff nurses from my previous visit who had been promoted. She had also gained responsibility for an extra ward as well which meant that I saw little or nothing of her.

This, I feel, was the first tangible sign I had seen of the decline of Britain's National Health Service, which was followed almost immediately by an even starker sign as I scrutinized my surroundings and was horrified to see some dried blood on the metalwork of my bed. This consequently drew my attention to the fact that the cleaners seemed to come round less frequently than before and had been transformed from a jolly bunch of West Indian women who always had a bit of a chat with you to a rather sullen group of malnourished-looking toughs who didn't even make eye contact, let alone cheer you up with a bit of banter.

However, it was not all bad news. Thankfully, as it would have been a touch embarrassing for both parties, the staff nurse who I had asked out for a date had moved on. Her replacement could not have been more different to the cool, highly professional, almost ice-queen persona I had fallen for. This one seemed to have modeled herself squarely (or roundly) on Baywatch. Busty as a barmaid, wearing plenty of make-up and barely regulation shoes, she tottered around the ward as though on her way home from a night-club. Her masterstroke was that she clearly, very clearly, wore the skimpiest of thongs – fire engine red – beneath her extremely tight, starched white uniform.

This may not sound too newsworthy today when we are accustomed to seeing all kinds of female underwear on display in the gaping void between crop top blouses and low-rise jeans, but this was in 1985 when thongs were almost unheard of outside of burlesque shows. I soon discovered that it was not just me who had spotted her lingerie preferences as nine other pairs of eyes slavishly followed her every move. Previously vigorous men would be suddenly struck incapable of sitting up in bed without her assistance; sure-handedness would be replaced by the fumbled dropping of books and pens as she walked past, the occupants hoping that she would bend down and retrieve the shower of objects hitting the floor. Just like the President thinks that all men talk into their shirt-cuffs, this nurse must have assumed that all men were clumsy, helpless, slavering oafs. But ward morale had never been higher; even the smoking room was empty when she was on duty.

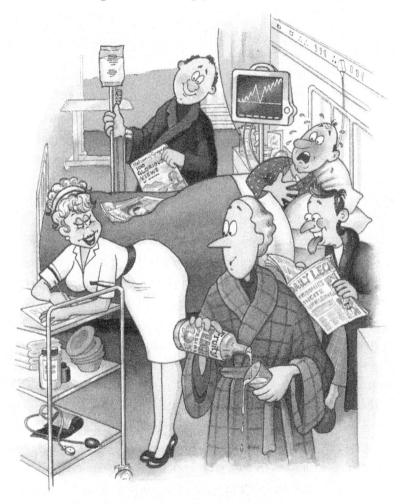

Thongs ain't what they used to be

Spurred on by the need to compare notes on this nursing phenomenon, I relented on my usual no-socializing rule and fell into conversation with two old-timers who had both contracted Crohn's disease decades ago. They were a couple of real, down-to-earth Birmingham guys who, once we got past the phwoaring about the nurse, seemed to take great delight in educating me as to what my future held.

"Had your kidney stones yet?" followed by a duet of noisy intakes of breath and a verdict of "Just you wait!" that was said with far too much relish for my liking. "Like passing broken glass!" "What about your ankylosing spondylitis, had any of that yet?"

And so it went on, each term getting more and more obscure-sounding but apparently all destined to become familiar to me. After an hour or so of medical clairvoyance, I retreated to my bed.

I broke my re-imposed silence when approached by a man, not much older than me, from the bed opposite who asked what I was in for. When I said my second operation for Crohn's, he gave a hollow, mirthless laugh and said that he was in for his thirteenth. Thirteenth! I was speechless. I can't remember what I mumbled in response but it was clear to me from his demeanor that he had given up, and who could blame him. He very obviously had no confidence that the thirteenth would be any more successful than the previous twelve.

I then kept an eye on any visits to his bed by his surgical team, which was a different one to mine, to pick up clues as to what was going on. I soon gathered the gist of the plot in that his last few operations, which seem to have happened pretty much without a pause, had not achieved the desired results with each operation getting increasingly complex and "heroic" in both duration and scope. I found it incredibly sad to see his wife, who dutifully visited every afternoon and evening, trying to keep his spirits up when he had nothing left in the tank. Wartime soldiers say that courage is not endless, each man having a finite supply, and I believe this to also be true about medical fortitude. We all have our limits.

It was quite apparent to me that here was a case where the medics had lost control of the poor guy's condition at some point and were resorting to ever more extreme measures. I was not surprised to hear about a year later that he had passed away, and it was a clear reminder that having an illness could turn out disastrously. If anything, the news spurred me on with my quest to retain as much control as possible over my illness and its treatment.

Tip #61: Avoid Becoming the Case They Lost Control Of

It is critical that you feel the specialists in charge of you and the surgeons on your case have some degree of control as to what is happening to your health. If you don't, then do everything in your power to be referred to someone else higher up the medical food chain. Too many medical disasters are caused by doctors refusing to admit they don't know what to do next.

Thankfully, I had none of these concerns as my operation, which was again performed by the maestro himself, passed off incident-free. This time, he informed me after the event, far from taking a conservative approach to what did or didn't constitute a stricture that needed plasty-ing, even the slightest narrowing had been subjected to the technique which, by this time, had made him a famous figure in the world of gastro-intestinal surgeons.

I was stunned to hear that he had performed nine stricture-plasties on me this time around. Coupled with the three I had had the first time, that equated to one for every two feet of small bowel.

"Was this some kind of record?" I asked him.

"In all likelihood," he replied.

His technique had been eagerly adopted by the surgical community and was already quite commonplace but, even so, I was probably now the world-record holder for number of strictureplasties. He had also since published his book on the subject and it did indeed have one of Cheryl's pictures of my insides in it. Fame at last.

Having had such a thorough re-boring of my small bowel, I was now confident that my blockage problems were all behind me. Dr. Ray popped by my bed and spent a good while giving me his perspective on the outcome. He confirmed that, as all the existing narrowings had been widened, then I should indeed be blockage-free, although it still might be a sensible precaution to remove from my diet the kinds of foods which were prone to getting stuck. This included, of course, mushrooms, in addition to sweet corn, peanuts and other firm items that could easily be inadvertently swallowed whole.

But the bigger thing on his mind was that being on steroids, while making me feel well, had clearly done nothing to prevent the formation of strictures. Given the well-documented risks of long-term steroid therapy, he proposed that this be gradually discontinued as the risks clearly outweighed the benefit of artificially induced high levels of appetite and energy. Once I was off them, we would, he informed me, try a range of other drug options that might help prevent any further strictures, as to have had twelve within the space of not even three years was almost unheard of. And on this sobering note, I returned home to commence another recuperation.

The Only Trouble With An Incurable Disease Is That It Doesn't Go Away

"'Tis not always in a physician's power to cure the sick; at times the disease is stronger than trained art."

— Ovid (Roman poet, 43 BC – AD 17)

AS WITH THE surgery, my recuperation was no longer a journey into the unknown as I felt that I was by now something of an expert. Since it was clear that my Crohn's was not a one-off event but was to be an endless cycle of remission, illness, drug regimes and surgery, I felt that I had to plan my recovery as part of a longer-term health-management strategy rather than merely trying to get well enough to return to work as soon as possible.

Tip #62: Take as Much Sick Leave for Recuperation as You Can Get

With Crohn's, you must take as much sick leave as your employer will tolerate. Once you return to work, they won't cut you any slack as they expect you are fully recovered and firing on all cylinders. It is much better to be absent for longer but be more effective when you return. You need to get as well as you possibly can to charge up your batteries before returning to the rigors of the workplace. If you do not, you are almost certainly just hastening your descent into your next health crisis and imperiling your continued employment.

But within this sick-leave philosophy, I did not believe that one should just laze around all day for the entire period. In my experience, the recovery process goes through several distinct phases, each requiring a slightly different recuperation strategy.

As soon as you get home, you are amazed at just how weak you feel – seemingly much weaker than you had been in hospital. This is because, in hospital, there is a small army of people who do absolutely everything for you. Once I had been home a few days, Audrey returned to work leaving me to fend for myself during the day. Even just making your own cups of coffee is a lot more than you were doing in hospital. So at this stage you need to do as little as possible.

The next phase kicks in a couple of weeks later when it dawns on you that you are feeling no stronger. You are just as exhausted at the end of the day as you were when you came out of hospital. Why don't you seem to be recovering? You worry that perhaps something has gone wrong. But this is, in fact, partly an illusion. As you imperceptibly recover, you unknowingly gradually increase the amount of effort you expend, not realizing that you are doing slightly more each day to reach the same level of exhaustion that sees you helpless on the sofa watching daytime TV when your partner returns. You feel you are making no progress because you are gauging your recovery on how exhausted you feel, not on how much you did to feel that way.

As your internal repair effort begins to wind down, you notice that you are feeling quite a lot better. As you have been feeling awful for so long, this phase can be quite euphoric. I would wake up feeling full of a latent energy that had been missing in my life for months. This is the most dangerous phase as you feel like you could go back to work, just for a couple of hours you tell yourself, keep yourself busy etc. Don't fall for it. Once you go back to work, it is impossible to ration it. Before you know it you will be expending more energy on work than your body is freeing up from its recovery process and then you will be short-changing your recovery. This isn't a case of maximizing time off work for its own sake – it's all part of being realistic and strategic about managing a long-term illness as well as a long-term career. In my case, when I could no longer tolerate resting while feeling energetic, I set myself a goal to redecorate the kitchen. Not all at once of course, but over many weeks, gradually doing more but always keeping my exertions behind the upward curve of my recovery.

Tip #63: Give Yourself a Project During Your Recovery

A home reno project is a part of the recovery process in that it helps you build up your stamina without the danger that you will be sucked back into the workplace too quickly. You have to be disciplined about not working too hard on the task. Pick something where you can keep control of how much time you spend on it and when you do the work.

My kitchen project work started off at maybe 10 minutes in a day, building up to a couple of hours a day as I got nearer my target return to work. I would then increasingly supplement the task with household work such as a bit of cleaning and cooking. It was during this second recovery period that I developed a lifelong love of planning an evening meal, going shopping for the ingredients and then cooking it. I still spent plenty of time reclining on the sofa reading books, newspapers and vegetating in front of daytime TV. When it came time to go back to work, I felt better than I had done for years and ready to make a real impact.

Tip #64: Make a Splash When You Return to Work

To have a successful career while having Crohn's, you have to add as much or more value in the reduced time you are in the workplace compared to your peers who have never taken a day's sick leave in their lives. You cannot do this if you are struggling because of still recovering from the effects of surgery and anesthesia. You want people thinking, "Thank goodness he's back, we've really missed his energy/enthusiasm/drive etc."

Initially, all seemed well and I viewed the future with my usual optimism. My appetite, while not gargantuan, had stabilized at a level that just about crept into the lower end of the "normal" range. I was able to lunch with my work colleagues without attracting comments on how little I ate, which I found a major relief.

Crohn's is, by its nature, a very personal illness in that most of the time you do not look ill at all to the outside world, even though you can go for very prolonged periods of feeling extremely unwell. The only real manifestations that can give you away are the frequency of your visits to the bathroom and the pathetically small amounts of food you consume while dining in public. Your friends and relatives who know you and your illness well tend to maintain a discreet silence while you are morosely pushing food round your plate. However, colleagues in the work canteen and waiters in restaurants always seem to succumb to the urge to pass comment. A jovial, "Off your food?" comment can get very tiresome when you hear it for the millionth time, and I have to fight the urge to bore the person into a coma with a 30-minute explanation as to why. Equally, when a waiter inevitably inquires, while collecting your plate of mostly untouched food, as to whether or not the food was

OK, I wish I could do better than, "Yes, it's me, I had a late breakfast."

But I was having a respite from such gastronomic interrogations as my appetite held up even while the steroids were slowly phased out such that, six months after the operation, I was off them completely. My optimism was boosted further by Doctor Ray booking me in for my next visit to the clinic, not four weeks later as had become the norm, but in the far-distant six months' time. Perhaps the corner really had been turned.

Or perhaps not. Gradually the old problems returned, but this time there was no benefit of the steroid rocket fuel to give me the illusion of still feeling well. I never did last the six months without clinic visits as I was back in Dr. Ray's office in August 1986 complaining of feeling as lively as a beached jellyfish with an appetite to match. He ordered another barium meal, the results of which in part vindicated my early return to the medical fray.

This time, the negatives on his light box showed not some obvious-looking strictures, but some fuzzy areas which he explained represented inflammation of the small bowel at its lower end. While not great news, he softened the blow by explaining that this should not cause me too much trouble in the way of symptoms as long as it was treated by putting me back on Metronidazole.

This plan proved even less successful than previous attempts to control my illness with non-steroid drugs. Even though I had taken it before, this time around I had to call a halt as it was giving me spells of nausea and dizziness. How can two courses of the same drug have differing effects on me, I wondered? No one knows, which to me is just more evidence that drug treatments are far less well understood than Big Pharma would have us all believe. It was at this stage that, in hindsight, the course of my illness entered the unknown as far as the medical profession was concerned.

The problem was that my symptoms at this stage – worsening appetite and energy levels coupled with a gradually increasing feeling of general crapness – were firstly very subjective. Secondly, they did not really fit with the mild-looking inflammation shown on the latest X-ray nor with the regular blood tests which, as I have explained previously, were not registering active inflammation. So by the beginning of 1987, I entered a phase where I wasn't receiving any treatment for what were a set of medically vague symptoms that were unsupported by any medically accepted evidence.

My appetite gradually diminished back to the levels of my sales force days and even beyond. Audrey would liquidize my meals so that I could perhaps get more nutrients into my body, but it was in vain. Let me tell you, when you have no appetite, liquidized lamb chops, potatoes and carrots (or any other main meal, as they all seemed remarkably similar when buzzed up) doesn't set the saliva glands gushing.

With the benefit of hindsight, it is at this point that I should have taken action to change specialist. The mismatch between my reported symptoms and what the tests were showing had become normal and, quite clearly, Dr. Ray was siding with the tests he knew so well, the corollary being that I must be either exaggerating or making myself so anxious that I was making myself feel ill. He never said this to me, but I later discovered in his letters to my family doctor that is exactly what he thought. I should have taken my business elsewhere, but I did not, and allowed things to drift along.

Tip #65: Don't Let Matters Drift
Always believe in yourself and seek a fresh pair of eyes unclouded by history if you feel you are not getting the treatment that your symptoms deserve.

However, I was not completely passive as, to supplement my by now inadequate diet, I began to treat the appetite and nutrition problem directly. I started on the fortified drinks one can buy in the health sections of food stores, and when these proved inadequate, my family doctor prescribed a pre-digested mix of all the nutrients a body needs. Known as an elemental diet, it was normally prescribed as a complete alternative to a regular diet, but in my case was additional to the few liquidized morsels I was managing to eat. It came in powder form which was then mixed with water and drunk during the day. I had to drink four pints each day, which was a huge effort as it looked, smelt and tasted like putrid swamp-water.

There is no doubt that this was a low point in my life. I was feeling terrible virtually all the time and eating had become an endurance rather than a pleasure. It is difficult when you can see no light at the end of the tunnel, but rather than sink into a black depression, I tried to focus myself on managing my diminished energy levels to at least remain productive at work. Audrey bore the brunt of this as I would be exhausted most evenings and not up to much socializing. But she was a rock for me to cling onto as she made sure that I could rest up as much as possible.

I soldiered on while feeling like this because I had convinced myself that I had submitted too early last time around when I had written to Dr. Ray demanding an operation. After all, here I was less than a year later feeling just as bad, if not worse than I had then, so where was the benefit of undergoing the trauma and risk of major surgery? This time, I told myself, I would tough it out as long as I possibly could before going under the knife again. But it was incredibly difficult. The diet took a Herculean effort to endure as it wasn't making me better; I was just getting worse more slowly than would have otherwise been the case. Thus my motivation to keep drinking the sludge was somewhat lacking.

Since nothing from the armory of modern medicine seemed to be doing me any good, it was at this point that I first turned to the world of alternative therapies. A colleague at work told me of a drink she had heard about that could apparently achieve marvelous results in people suffering from Crohn's disease. The drink in question was called Aloe Vera. Before jumping into this new world, I once again trotted off down to the reference library to do my due diligence.

You may have come across Aloe Vera, as had I, as something listed amongst the ingredients of your shampoo. It has also been known to appear in cosmetics, moisturizers, soaps and even infused into facial tissues. This was not a promising start as something to drink. However, it did have a long track record of usage in herbal medicines, having been mentioned in ancient Egyptian papyri, Greek and Roman texts, and it even pops up in the Bible, "And there came also Nicodemus, which at the first came to Jesus by night, and brought a mixture of myrrh and aloes..." (John 19:39-40). As good a celebrity endorsement as one could wish for, although whether Jesus drank the stuff, as I was supposed to, or merely washed his hair with it is not made clear.

It turned out that this allegedly miracle drink could only be bought through a kind of pyramid-selling scheme, and my colleague knew someone who knew someone who was selling the stuff, so was able to procure me a gallon bottle. I have to say it was so awful that it made the elemental diet taste divine. This was seriously unpalatable stuff. But anyway, needs must so I forced myself to drink my way through the gallon. When it came time to order another, I was invited along to the local branch meeting of the Aloe Vera sellers' organization, which was a real eye-opener.

I have never been to a revivalist religious meeting, but this event was exactly how I had pictured one. There were about twenty people in attendance who seemed to be the boots-on-the-ground sales force for this one product. The meeting was led by a regional manager, whose overwhelming passion for the miracles of Aloe Vera was no doubt fuelled by the fact he was getting a fat cut of every bottle sold by all these people in the pyramid underneath him. He would chant out the various lines of sales patter for Aloe Vera, which would be repeated by a swaying, almost hypnotic audience.

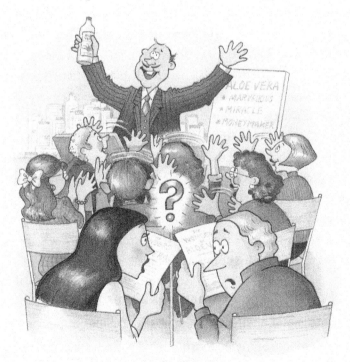

The alternative medicine scene

It was all very spooky. The worst bit came when he stopped the chanting and uttered those words dreaded by new congregants everywhere,

"..and I believe we have a new member with us today.."

After taking the obligatory round of applause and dodging the multiple requests to become an evangelist/seller for the stuff, Audrey and I beat a hasty retreat.

I never touched a drop of it again, my reasoning being that, if this really was either a miracle cure or at least an effective treatment for Crohn's disease, then surely, since it had been around since the time of Jesus, it would have been on prescription by now rather than being sold like Tupperware. The next time I went into the Ward 8 clinic, I mentioned I had been taking this stuff and the response of the medic was as if I had said I had been taking strychnine mixed with cow dung.

Medics, in my experience, never ever respond well to a conversation about alternative therapies. Some, so as not to appear too out-of-touch, will preface their contribution with some platitude about them probably not doing any harm, but you will be made to feel like a superstitious throwback from the witch-burning era. I suppose they must take it as a bit of a slap in the face when you say you are going to go for some unscientific approach.

Tip #66: Going Alternative is Better Than Nothing

Dabbling in alternative therapies is a matter of personal preference. But, if modern medicine has run out of options, which it had for me, then even the feeling of trying to do something useful is better for morale than impotently and mutely suffering on. Do not let medical disdain deter you from trying to contribute to your own well-being, no matter how bizarre the remedy. Personally, I would drink monkey

pee while naked in the middle of Sunday Mass if I thought
it might be doing me even the slightest amount of good.

The only good news at this time was that I was still managing to be
effective at work despite being far from the top of my game. This
was because my choice to move into marketing Cadbury's seasonal
product ranges was proving to be an even better decision than I had
first imagined.

Prior to my taking the role, it had been the Cinderella job in the
department. The previous two incumbents had been given the job
almost as a penalty for not having delivered in other roles, both
staying in the role only about a year before leaving the company.
This meant that senior management's expectations for the job had
been reduced, which worked for me as I was able to build a level of
knowledge and competence well beyond what they had come to
expect in the role, which compensated for a level of sick leave well
above the department average.

Tip #67: Look for Jobs That Have Been Undervalued in the Past

You can still be ambitious while putting your health first. It
is a matter of looking further ahead than your peers and
making more thoughtful career choices where you get your
next promotion.

I had taken the decision not to share anything more than the
minimum with my employer about my thoughts on developing my
career within the constraints of illness. This was simply because I
did not want my illness to become a workplace issue. By taking a
role where the company had quite modest expectations of what
could be achieved, I was able, even when quite ill, to exceed those

expectations. I am not sure that I could have achieved this effect if I had openly shared my strategy with them beforehand.

Back in the Ward 8 clinic, the one piece of hard evidence that broke through Dr. Ray's skepticism was that I was still losing weight, despite the efforts I was making on my own behalf to maintain my nutrition. So, in April 1988, a mere nine months after the last one, I was, once again, dispatched for another Super Slurpee-sized dose of barium, illuminated by another five years' worth of radiation.

It was becoming obvious by this point that my life with Crohn's would be accompanied by plentiful visits to the medical imaging department as medics love to see what's going on inside the digestive tract. For this, they have Wilhelm Roentgen to thank. Wilhelm was a German physicist who, on November 8, 1895, discovered X-rays by complete accident. He was experimenting with the newly invented cathode ray tube which, in one test, he covered up completely with black cardboard in a darkened room before switching it on. Having previously ensured his cardboard cover allowed no light to escape the tube, he was stunned to see in the gloom a shimmering over on his workbench. Investigation revealed the shimmering to be coming from a screen coated in barium platinocyanide he was intending to use for another test.

Realizing that this was some previously undiscovered type of radiation, he conducted further experiments that included, a mere two weeks after his initial discovery, taking the first-ever X-ray image, this being of his wife's hand. Upon seeing the outline of her finger bones, she apparently exclaimed, "I have seen my own death!" Given that both Roentgen and his laboratory assistant would later succumb to radiation poisoning, she had in fact seen their deaths rather than her own. Roentgen was a modest chap who resisted patenting his discovery as he wanted it to be available to all and even gave away the money that came with his Nobel Prize. His lasting fame is that units of dosage of X-rays (a term he coined) are measured in Roentgens.

My reason for telling you all this is that, by now, my Roentgen account was most definitely running quite high, evidenced by my X-ray folder now bulging more than two inches thick with accumulated negatives. This latest set of Roentgen-rays showed what Dr. Ray described as "minor mucosal changes of Crohn's disease but not enough to give him the symptoms he describes". Business as usual then. To look like something was being done, I was put back on Asacol, but as usual, it achieved nothing.

The next six months went by as my own version of Groundhog Day. Repeated visits to Dr. Ray; repeated reassurances that the blood tests were normal, and all the while accompanied by a gradual, almost imperceptible decline in my appetite, my weight, my feeling of well-being and my confidence that I was ever going to feel better. Six months later, in September 1988, the log-jam was finally broken when yet another barium meal showed not just the minor stuff of the last two, but what Dr. Ray described to my family doctor as "extensive jejunal disease with stricture formation". This came as a complete surprise to everyone involved, and should have raised some questions as to the efficacy of the blood tests which I had been having as regularly as clockwork and which had shown nothing amiss.

The surprise was twofold, the first being the location of this latest outbreak. Jejunal disease refers to inflammation in the part of the small bowel known as the jejunum. This is the upper part of the small bowel, immediately after where the stomach has handed things over to the duodenum, and constitutes about 40% of the overall length of the small bowel, the remainder being called the ileum. My previous two surgeries had been involved exclusively in dealing with strictures in the ileum, so this now meant that my entire small bowel was stricken to some degree or other. The second surprise, at least for Dr. Ray and his crew, was the extent of the inflammation, given that their precious tests had been showing nothing really amiss.

Of course, this meant another encounter with the scalpel, the prospect of which took my eye off what should have been a detailed inquest into how all this inflammation had come about, finishing with a Perry Mason-like conclusive proof that I had been right all along.

At this stage, I should have forced the issue as to why precedence was being given to blood tests at the expense of my reported symptoms, when it was now clear that the blood work was, at least in my case, functionally useless in recording the progress of the Crohn's. I wish I had done so, but I think the relief on getting some proper treatment put it from my mind. If I had brought this up, the outcome would have been a realization that I was in fact an accurate symptom-reporter rather than some depressive hypochondriac.

Tip #68: Don't be Afraid to Ask the Difficult Questions

Don't make my mistake: When you have real evidence that would change the medics' perception of how to manage your case, bring it up and force the issue, no matter how difficult the conversation might be.

So in November 1988, almost three years since my last surgery, most of which had been passed feeling terrible, I went in once again for another appointment with the master strictureplasterer.

Nothing dramatic happened during the surgery and by now the operations were all beginning to blend into one in my mind anyway.

I was becoming used to them as a feature of my life rather than them being novel events. However, this time he departed from his track record of just doing regular strictureplasties on me and, in addition to three more of the kind I was world record holder in, gave me two of what are called Finney Strictureplasties. These were an elongated version that dealt with strictures too close to each other to be done separately, a recognition of just how badly inflamed my jejunum had become.

There was, however, a novel and unwelcome aspect to the immediate post-operative period. As I gradually emerged from the blackness and came round from the anesthetic, my first sensation was not the usual intense throbbing of the recently slashed and sewn abdomen, but a really sharp pain in my right eye. Once I had recovered the powers of speech, I complained long and loud to Audrey and my mother, the latter of whom went off in a determined frame of mind to lasso a senior member of the surgical team and have this unlikely post-operative symptom diagnosed and resolved.

Helpless against the irresistible force that is my mother's maternal urge to protect her young on her own turf, the second-in-command meekly put in an appearance and soon ascertained that the problem was a deep scratch to my eyeball. Eh? How had that happened? Once again, the code of medical omertà swung in to action. While all agreed the conceptual cause as being that something or someone must have scratched it during the process of taping my eyes shut – a process that happens after you have been anaesthetized and while the surgeon is still scrubbing his fingernails – of course, no one was held to account. If that had been in America, I could have sued for zillions.

The solution was the numbing of my eyeball with some drops which meant I had to wear an eye-patch to reduce the chance of me inadvertently causing even more damage to an eyeball now completely devoid of feeling. As if I needed any further evidence that, for the most part, hospitals and surgeries are dangerous and best avoided.

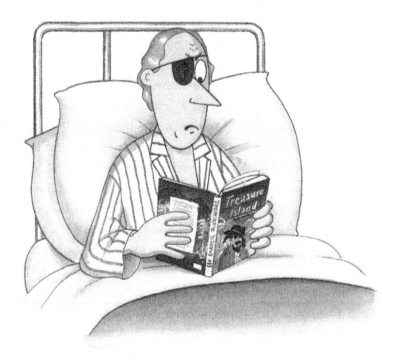

Patched up

No End In Sight

"Physicians and politicians resemble one another in this respect: that some defend the constitution and others destroy it."

— Anon

HAVING ESCAPED FROM the hospital with no other serious injuries, this time during my recovery period I planned and gradually implemented a back yard landscaping of the new house we had recently moved into. After an uneventful recuperation and the building of a paved area that would outlast the pyramids, I returned to work in my seasonal role. Both the company and I had now got used to my absences and I was able to pick up where I had left off.

But, within a matter of a few months, the disease, which of course had never gone away, was once again making its presence known to me. This time I would be treated to one of the rarer symptoms associated with Crohn's, a perianal fistula, or, to put it more bluntly, a second butt-hole. This sounds like something that could only happen to Bart Simpson but is not as completely disgusting as one might imagine.

It all relates back to my perianal abscesses of the past. Sometimes, when a gland deep in the nether regions becomes infected, rather than manifest itself in an excruciating abscess due to the build-up of pus, it tries to solve the problem itself by tunneling its way towards the open air. On the odd occasion it accomplishes this feat, the outcome is a very narrow passage from the gland to the skin near the rear end. Since the same gland has its own opening into the anal canal, it has, in effect, created a county road diversion to the outside world from the interstate highway that is the anal canal.

I first became aware of this alternate exit by an intense itch which, given its location, proved extremely difficult to attend to during work hours without attracting disapproving glances. On the odd occasions when other attendees at meetings had their attentions fixed on the screen, I would have a surreptitious scratch, or, failing that, a good shifting around on my chair, but all to no avail. This was an itch that could not be scratched into submission.

However, the itching became the least of my problems as, when the tunneling finally broke surface, the outcome was a passage between my digestive system and the outside world that had no muscles by which to control it. This meant that, while a tight clenching of the buttocks could be usually counted on to keep a good fart in check until circumstances allowed its release, in my case a tiny amount could bypass the road-block with me being helpless to stop it. Although this could have made me into a seemingly shameless and socially unaware serial farter, fortunately the passage was so narrow that it only allowed for a tiny squeak that could easily be mistaken for a passing mouse or someone leaning back on an office chair.

While this development panicked me somewhat, once I had read up about it I felt reassured that it was not the beginning of a collapse of my normal bodily functions. Fistulas, once they appear, tend to remain constant in size and scope and are, in many cases, better left alone. Since I was spared the very occasional manifestation of this alternate route being able to pass stools, the only thing I had to deal with was that it leaked a tiny, but consistent stream of moisture produced by the gland. This meant that I had to take to wearing female panty-liners, the only risk being that I would absentmindedly put one in on the days when I would be playing football and risk raised eyebrows in the manly world of the dressing room. Otherwise, my health, while far from perfect, was somewhat better than had been the case prior to the previous operation, so things carried on uneventfully for 10 months or so until I was back again in Ward 8 complaining of more abdominal pain. A prescription for more Asacol was the result and, when this proved to be ineffective, I was put on a new drug called Pentasa. This was just basically the same ingredient but chemically packaged so that it was only released within the small bowel, bathing the sides, rather than being absorbed in the stomach like most other drugs and working via the bloodstream. But same drug, same non-result.

The outcome was now depressingly predictable and another barium meal in January 1991 confirmed the inevitable. More strictures had appeared and the only solution was more strictureplasties. Once inside me, in addition to plastying the strictures, the surgeon took the decision to remove a 10cm segment that had been one of the longer strictureplasties he had done the last time as apparently it wasn't looking too good. Ah well, it had been worth a try, or so I thought at the time.

I cannot deny that, at this point, my morale was low. There just seemed to be no end to it. But sometimes there isn't a course of treatment that will work and then you just have to suck it up without getting too depressed.

Tip #69: Keep Looking Forward to Better Times

Keep a positive frame of mind that there are new therapies and surgical techniques being developed all the time and that your current malaise will not last forever.

Four major abdominal operations within the space of eight years no doubt seems like a lot and you may be asking if there was not any alternative. I don't think the problem was that the surgeon was trigger-happy. His philosophy was, "Don't operate until a patient gets a complication from Crohn's disease; but don't wait for the complication to get more complicated", a mantra that was accepted as best practice in the area and one I found difficult to argue with. Meanwhile, the physician had no treatments that were capable of stopping my Crohn's from creating strictures. Steroids hadn't stopped it and neither had any of the other drugs I had been prescribed. The fact is that medical science has its limits and sometimes there is not a lot anyone can do about it.

During this latest recovery from surgery, I had not thought beyond going back into my seasonal marketing job that I still thoroughly enjoyed and was still being successful at. But around four weeks prior to my planned re-entry date, my boss approached me with a proposition that came completely from left field. Not long before I had gone in for this latest surgery, Cadbury had opened a visitor centre on their main factory site. It had been a massive investment by the company, some $12 million, to try and recreate the benefits of the long-defunct factory tours. However, it had not got off to a good start and my boss, who was ultimately responsible for it, had decided that it needed a fresh perspective in its management. What is more, he had decided that I was the man for the job.

Once I had got over the shock of being offered a new job, I came to the realization that, while the seasonal job still checked all the boxes, I should not and could not stay there forever. I had been in the role for six years, which is a lifetime in a marketing role, and had been promoted twice within it, but there would undoubtedly come a point when success would inevitably wane and then I would risk being stigmatized as the useless old-timer in the corner. Also, in truth, this new job offer excited me much more than the prospect of a return to running the seasonal portfolio.

This Cadbury World job was very clearly a fix-it-and-move-on posting, for which the timing was perfect. I would be feeling as well and as energetic as I ever did during the first few months back at work and then who knows? If I stayed feeling well there could easily be another such role with the chance to make another quick and visible impact or, if I succumbed again, I was confident I could get the job done at Cadbury World and then move onto a more sedate role where I could shelter while still doing a good job for the company. It also met my criteria of being a job where there existed a strong possibility of being able to exceed expectations, due to the poor start the venture had encountered. So, somewhat impulsively, since I had no idea what would be involved in running a visitor centre that attracted 350,000 people a year and employed 120 staff, I said yes.

It would have been very easy to pass on this opportunity and to play safe by staying in a job where I was very comfortable. But, by this point, I had been through enough surgeries to know I would have at least a year of feeling well enough to be capable of firing on all cylinders in the workplace. A year in this job, if successful, would be a far bigger contributor in convincing the company I was worth persevering with than a seventh year in my old job.

Tip #70: Sometimes You Have to Go For It.

While, with Crohn's, you have to be much more risk aware in your career planning, that does not mean you should always be risk averse. You don't want to spend your life resentful at how the illness has held you back.

This turned out to be a very smart career move but that came with a trade-off in my health. In the beginning, although it was much harder work than I was used to, I was feeling more energetic than I had for most of the previous eight years. It was also the first job in my career that was essentially one of managing rather than doing. I found that the disciplines I had taught myself about working smarter paid dividends in this new role. Giving direction to my team of managers, making decisions and being visible and accessible to the employees seemed to come easier to me because of the work habits I had adopted to make up for my previous absences.

Over the next twelve months, the management team and I managed to turn the enterprise around and resolve just about all the issues that had been attracting the complaints. But the fact that it was much harder work than I was used to definitely speeded up my by now inevitable decline in health. Towards the end of 1992, a mere eighteen months after I had returned to work from the last surgery, I was already in bad shape. Fortunately, by this time, Cadbury World was running much more smoothly so I was still able to do a reasonable job while running at well under full capacity.

But I was perturbed by a very unwelcome change to my usual set of symptoms. While I had been used to diarrhea as a regular feature of my life, I had been stricken by outpouring of such virulence, unpleasantness and longevity that I thought it could only have come from the Devil's own bottom. It was also accompanied by flatulence that went far beyond the imaginable in terms of both quantity and repulsiveness. I could have filled the Hindenburg airship on a daily basis while asphyxiating its passengers and crew.

These were by far the most stressful symptoms I had endured to date because of the social aspect. I could keep pain to myself. Poor appetite could be quite stressful when in a social situation as I have described previously. But with this diarrhea and flatulence, virtually any social gathering was a source of great stress to me. If I kept it bottled up I would soon be in intense discomfort as the horrible aroma meant that subtle lettings off were impossible and frequent trips to the john soon began raising eyebrows. Plus, I was always at risk of butt number two going rogue. Conversely, if I let the farts out, then I would soon be branded a social outcast.

These new symptoms went on for months on end but, each time I mentioned them in the Ward 8 clinic, they were brushed off as being just temporary inconveniences of the illness. After a couple of clinics like this, I eventually cracked and forcefully explained that I knew what diarrhea and flatulence were like, but these symptoms were completely out of the ordinary and were basically ruining my life. To get Dr. Ray's full attention, I made it clear that I was not going to leave his office until he took these symptoms seriously and ordered up some tests. It was at this point I realized the power of the immovable patient – perhaps something I had learned from the professional complainers who felt comfortable poking me in the chest while ranting away at Cadbury World.

Tip #71: Dig Your Feet in Now and Again

Patients who ignore all cues from the medic that their allotted time is up and keep on about whatever is bothering them will probably get what they want because the efficiency of a busy clinic is imperiled. The medic would rather do what you want and get you out than have the clinic get completely backlogged by your intransigence. Use this ploy very sparingly, only when you are in real dire straits. It's the contrast to your normal demeanor that hits home with the medic. Do not use it to cry wolf or you will never be taken seriously.

As a consequence of my General Custer impression in his office, in addition to the ordering of a stool sample test, a barium meal was also booked for a few weeks' time.

Prior to the barium meal, I was back again at the clinic in late December 1992 to get the results of the stool sample. It did indeed confirm that I was infested by enormous amounts of an unusual bacteria, so I was prescribed antibiotics and then ushered on my way by the random medic I saw. A couple of days later, my parents came to visit us for New Year and, when I opened the front door, my mother reacted as though she had seen a ghost. This was because I was paler than she had ever seen me before. She immediately insisted that I book to see the family doctor who, because of our good relationship, saw me the same day.

His initial response was that I looked massively anemic and he ordered up an immediate blood test. I had to take it myself to the blood clinic at the local hospital, this being New Year's Eve which meant that the normal process would take days. Later that afternoon, he phoned me to say the results were in and that he had arranged for me to go into Ward 8 for an immediate blood transfusion, which, since I was exceptionally anemic, would likely involve an overnight stay. So I packed a bag, phoned for a taxi and left Audrey to entertain my parents. Thus, I spent the evening and night of New Year's Eve, 1992, sitting in a bed in hospital being given four units of blood. Happy New Year.

Apparently I had been so short of the stuff the doctor was amazed that I was still walking around. Even the transfusion did not go smoothly as my temperature rocketed up to 104 while I was receiving the third bag. It eventually came back down and when I quizzed the doctor about it, she said that blood contains all sorts of things that can upset your own body's defenses. I then spent the rest of the night with visions of syphilitic, drug-addled hobos having sold the blood that was dripping steadily into my veins.

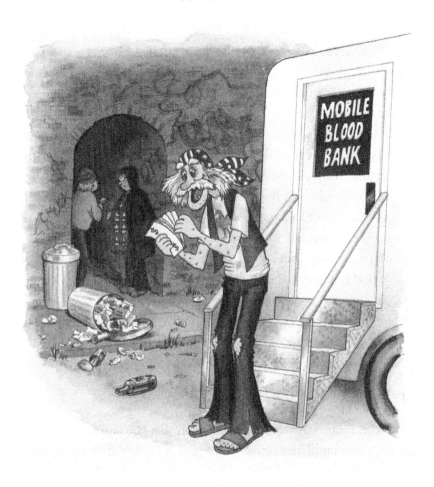

Blood brother

My vampire appearance had come about because, with active Crohn's disease, you can lose blood from an inflamed portion of your bowel and not notice that you are doing so if the inflammation is high up in your system. By the time the blood comes out it is indistinguishable from your motions, which largely consist of dead blood cells anyway. When I returned home next day, my mother was shocked to hear that I had been in the Ward 8 clinic only a couple of days earlier and that my anemia had not been spotted. This prompted her, first thing on January 2nd, to call Dr. Ray personally to lecture him on the abject inefficiency of whichever doctor had seen me.

One of the drawbacks of a specialist clinic is that sometimes doctors can be so specialized that anything that does not fit with their standard check list of symptoms gets ignored. They treat a very specialized condition rather than the whole patient. Because I had not complained of losing blood, the fact that I was deathly pale had simply not registered. And by seeing a different doctor from a month previously, there was not the opportunity for someone to notice that my appearance had changed.

Tip #72: Try to Keep Seeing the Same Doctor

Try, whenever possible, to see the same specialist from one visit to the next. There are benefits to continuity in that they might be able to recall you from your last visit.

However, there was some good news in that the antibiotics had a dramatic and immediate effect on me, killing the guilty bacteria that had been lurking in and around the various nooks and crannies of my small bowel that had been created by my previous surgeries. But that was it for good news. As the barium meal was looming, I began 1993 on another starvation diet.

The barium meal confirmed that I needed to go in for my fifth bout of surgery in less than 10 years. The time span from the last surgery was the shortest yet, a mere 23 months. At this stage I really did wonder what the future held for me and whether I would ever reach the age of 40. The symptoms were worse than ever and the reoccurrences more frequent than ever. Where would it all end? Would I simply run out of bowel before things settled down? Dr. Ray tried to reassure me that, although my case had been unusually severe, the usual trend in Crohn's disease was that it would settle down as the patient entered middle age. Since there seemed no sign whatsoever of any settling down, I took that with a pinch of salt.

The subsequent surgical stay in Ward 8 was the least inspiring to date. My usual surgeon had retired and been replaced by what seemed to me an exceptionally bad-tempered female surgeon who had the staff literally quaking in terror. Not that I was too bothered about the staff, which seemed to be largely made up of an ever-changing roster of agency nurses who knew less about Crohn's disease than I did. Just to cap it all off, the hospital was being closed and merged with another, allegedly as an efficiency measure, and Ward 8 was closing the week after I was due to leave. People were unscrewing and carting away fixtures and fittings while I was there.

On this last stay in Ward 8, for once I struck up a conversation with the man in the next bed who was also a Crohn's sufferer and in for a similar operation to mine. He was a charming and amusing old chap, well into his seventies, who had me transfixed with tales of how, when he was a teen, he had played soccer on the same team as Tommy Lawton. Just so you understand the significance of this, Tommy had been the 1930s equivalent of David Beckham in terms of fame.

But, although I enjoyed chatting to the old boy, I found the experience fundamentally depressing. Would I, I asked myself, still be going through these surgeries when I was his age? Would the rest of my life consist of short periods of relative good health that would be mere occasional oases in an otherwise endless desert of illness, stressful symptoms and surgeries? It was not an attractive prospect and one I tried hard to put out of my mind.

The post-game report on my surgery from the scary surgeon mainly highlighted the removal of the second Finney strictureplasty that had been done two operations ago. It turned out that this had become effectively a blind loop in my bowel that had harbored the bacteria which had been the source of my diabolical farts. Although I had eventually been prescribed antibiotics that did kill the bacteria, because the loop was always a safe haven for them, they had soon returned along with their horrible effects.

Because the Finney technique had been very new when used on me, this side effect of it was unknown at the time. Thus, the doctors didn't recognize my appalling symptoms as fitting within the accepted symptoms of my Crohn's and had therefore airily dismissed me as just another patient complaining about a bit of gas. My attempts to describe my gas and diarrhea as being far beyond the bounds of normality had fallen on deaf ears because normal gas and diarrhea are features of Crohn's, so the assumption must have been that I was exaggerating. More damned hoof-beats!

Of course, this raises the question of whether or not you should sign up for new treatments if you can also be subject to new symptoms which will most likely not register with one-track-mind specialists.

New treatments can bring unheralded relief compared to existing options but it is clear, at least to me, that I would have been better off without the Finney strictureplasties as there is no doubt they made my quality of life significantly worse. But, on the other hand, I had been a very early recipient of the original strictureplasty technique, which I am in no doubt radically improved my prospects compared to the option of cutting all the strictures out. I would have run out of bowel years ago. So these things can cut both ways.

Tip #73: Is There a Fall-back Plan?

You should make the judgment as to whether or not to sign up for new treatments and/or procedures based on three criteria: how desperate you are for relief; a thorough understanding as to the limitations of existing options, and what the fall-back plan is if the new innovations don't work.

I would have been delighted if this had been the only negative impact I was to suffer from my treatment during the long course of my illness up to this point. But unfortunately there are unintended consequences to any medical intervention in the workings of your body, of which I ended up having more than my fair share.

Collateral Damage

"The worst thing about medicine is that one kind makes another necessary."

> **— Elbert Hubbard (American writer and philosopher 1856 – 1915)**

AS I HAVE previously described, until the onset of the first symptoms of Crohn's disease in my late teens, I had been a very healthy person. But, as I went through my twenties and thirties, I accumulated such an array of medical problems that I turned into someone who was a good candidate for being invited to the family doctor's office Christmas party. It actually took many years for it to dawn on me that I was still, apart from my Crohn's, a basically healthy person.

Everything else I was to suffer from was either an indirect symptom of the Crohn's or a direct consequence of one of the treatments. There were Crohn's-related events that I did not report, as I did not know they were related. There were impacts of the drugs I was taking – particularly the steroids – that were treated as being quite separate events. And there were impacts of the X-ray investigations that were to nearly kill me.

Tip #74: Assume It's Connected Until Proven Otherwise

If the same happens to you, where after you have been diagnosed with Crohn's you switch from never seeing a doctor for anything to seeing a host of them for all sorts of things, always assume until proven otherwise that every new medical event is connected to either the investigation, treatment or course of your main complaint. Report all events, no matter how unrelated they seem, to the gastro-enterologist and your family doctor.

The first such event in my case was one that I did not report to the Ward 8 crowd at the time as it seemed completely unconnected to my Crohn's. In June 1987, Audrey and I had gone on holiday to the Austrian Alps. We would take the chairlift up the mountain and then enjoy the many different walks back to the town. The meadows were lush and green, populated by contented brown and white cows, the bells around their necks clanking away with that marvelous alpine sound. One almost expected hosts of dancing children to appear from behind every barn, yodeling merrily away.

On one such walk, we went off the beaten track to see a water-fall where the route back involved us clambering down some quite steep rocks. While Audrey took the less steep longer route around, I leapt off a large overhang about three feet high onto the ground below and, on landing, felt an intense pain in my left knee. I must confess I did not execute a textbook Green Beret roll, but even so, as I had grown up in the country and spent a large part of my childhood playing in a local disused stone quarry, I was well used to incurring slight twists and sprains, so I had no doubt this was just a tweak that could be easily walked off.

However, far from walking it off, the pain became increasingly intense, to the point where the only way I could make any forward progress at all was to walk sideways, dragging my left leg along, and we were still miles away from our village or indeed any signs of human habitation at all. Of course, in those days, there were no mobile phones to summon help, so I leaned on Audrey's shoulder and we just had to plod on at the pace of Antarctic explorers dragging 2000lb sleds. Indeed, at one point, when I really thought I could go no further, I asked Audrey to leave me by the wayside and carry on herself. But she would have none of it and we eventually crawled back to our hotel.

Over the next few days, the knee eased a little and it seemed to have been just a bad sprain, so I did not mention it to any doctor when we returned. But this knee was to trouble me for years afterwards, hurting intensely for a couple of days after playing soccer and occasionally giving way as I was making some innocuous maneuver. It became normal for me to randomly collapse while stepping onto the escalator in department stores.

It wasn't until 1997 that the mystery was solved when, while running on a treadmill — ironically during the taking of an obligatory company medical — my knee locked completely. This finally prompted me to mention it to the family doctor, who sent me to see a knee specialist. A set of X-rays was organized that showed quite clearly that a large chunk of bone, about the size of a walnut, had broken away from one of the two "knuckles" that make up the bottom of the femur, and had been floating around in my knee all this time until finally and irrevocably getting stuck.

When the specialist quizzed me about how this might have come about, the only explanation that made any sense to him was that, on this walking holiday, the bone had cracked and then, over the years, eventually become detached. He was mystified as to how jumping down three feet could cause such damage until I mentioned that I had, in the years prior, been on high doses of steroids. All then became clear to him because one of the most potent side effects of steroids is thinning of the bones. So I had to undergo yet another general anesthetic while he opened up my knee, removed the offending bone, and did his best to mitigate the damage done to the femur. His parting shot was that, while the knee would feel fine for the time being, I was guaranteed to have future problems with it in middle age and beyond. Marvelous.

I am now middle-aged and can report that he was a competent predictor: Even though I have long since stopped playing soccer and running to avoid further impact damage, the knee randomly swells up from time to time. Will it last me out or will I need a knee transplant? Nobody knows, but one thing I am sure of is that, if I had not been on steroids, I would not have a seriously damaged knee.

Tip #75: Medical Treatment is ALWAYS About Trade-offs; There are No Free Rides

It is a mistake to assume that you are getting completely unbiased advice from a specialist: They spend their working lives immersed in your main complaint but next to no time dealing with the unintended consequences of the treatment. They will always, in my experience, strongly recommend the best single treatment for the specific symptoms under discussion, despite the potential side effects or risk of subsequent issues. Your family doctor can be a good point of reference as you consider treatment options – they deal with everything so might have a more balanced view.

The next seemingly random medical event in my life came during the period I was being prescribed a series of antibiotics. My family doctor had a policy of not OK-ing by phone any and every request for repeat prescriptions, but having regular review consultations with me. At the time, I had not yet appreciated how best to fit the family doctor into my various strategies for dealing with Crohn's, so

I viewed these consultations as largely a waste of time for both of us. However, I dutifully went along to them all as they did not seem to do me any great harm.

In one of these catch-ups, after we had gone through the latest updates he had received from Dr. Ray, he finished off as usual with a polite, "Is there anything else?" At that precise moment, I could feel an itch in the area of an innocuous-looking mole on my chest. This mole, which had been there for as long as I could remember, had recently begun to itch intermittently and had also changed slightly in that there was what looked like a tiny bit of sunburn-type skin peeling around its circumference. Since he was asking the question at the precise moment it was itching, I mentioned it. He had a close look, announced that it looked insignificant, then asked if I wanted to get it looked at by a dermatologist. I prevaricated as it wasn't like I didn't go into hospitals enough already, but decided, since I had been the one to raise the issue, I might as well follow the process through. So he booked me in to see the dermatologist at the local hospital.

A couple of weeks later, the specialist had a good look at it through his magnifying glass, announced that it looked perfectly normal to him, then asked if I wanted him to remove it. Again, I hesitated before agreeing, swayed by his offer to do it immediately. So, after a surprisingly painful jab of local anesthetic, he used a hole-punch kind of device to cut it out and off it went to the lab to be analyzed, with me being booked to come back in another couple of weeks for the results.

When I came back, my medical radar sprang into action the second I was ushered into his office as he avoided eye contact. He was also a bit of a mumbler, so I struggled to follow what he was saying until I was electrified by the phrase, "malignant melanoma".

"What?????" I almost shouted.

Then he repeated more slowly and clearly the findings that, inside the mole, was a malignant melanoma in its early stages. It had not yet penetrated through the entirety of the various layers of skin, so the chances were that it had not yet spread. But these melanomas were the worst kind of skin cancer and one could never be too sure.

That being the case, he sprang into immediate action, removing a much larger piece of tissue surrounding the mole site and sending me down the corridor for a blood test and chest X-ray to check for signs that the cancer had not spread. He also announced that I would be coming back to see him on a regular basis for the next five years, after which, if I was still alive, I would be given the official all-clear. When I came back a week later for the results of the tests, which were thankfully clear, he left me in no doubt that this had been a lucky escape.

"I had a guy like you in just last week, with a similar benign-looking mole, but he had left it three months longer than you and there is nothing we can do for him. Finito."

A bit like after almost being involved in a car crash where you keep going over in your mind, "What if?", I could not stop thinking about the unlikely sequence of events that led to the mole being removed when it had been. What if I hadn't been seeing the family doctor on a regular basis? What if the mole hadn't been itching at that precise moment? What if I had turned down the offer to get it looked at? Or removed? At that moment, I felt like the luckiest man alive.

Tip #76: Never Put Off Seeing a Doctor

It is very common to put off going to the doctor, perhaps due to hoping that whatever it is will go away, or not wanting to "bother the doctor", or perhaps a fear of what might be involved. These are all big mistakes. Do not hesitate to

> go to the doctor. The possible consequences of waiting too
> long are simply not worth it.

After doing my usual homework in the reference library, I calculated the chances of the same person contracting both Crohn's disease AND a malignant melanoma as being forty-eight million to one, i.e., I was in all likelihood the only person in Britain to have contracted both if they were independent events, which was the assumption at the time. The dermatologist had gone through the standard checklist for melanoma sufferers: fair hair/skin, blue eyes, office job and had been burnt to a crisp on a few two-week holidays in Spain. I was a textbook case as far as he was concerned.

However, there was a connection with my Crohn's that, once again, only became apparent many years later, in 2008 to be precise. I noticed a strange mark on my lower back where the skin felt slightly rough. I had this removed and the tests showed that it was a basal cell carcinoma. However, the dermatologist I saw second time around could not believe that I had suffered from two skin cancers, both occurring on the trunk of my body. Apparently, he informed me, this would only ever happen to someone who spent large parts of the day shirtless in the sunshine: construction workers, surfer dudes, that kind of thing. For an office worker, it made no sense at all, especially when I informed him that I had not once taken my shirt off in the sunshine since the day the melanoma had been diagnosed nearly twenty years earlier.

The solution to this mystery came when I informed him just how many barium meals and barium enemas I had undergone since being diagnosed – I could recall ten. These examinations, particularly in the earlier years before technology improved, had subjected me to massive doses of radiation. One barium meal equated to the same radiation as over two hundred chest X-rays, a month spent in space or five years' worth of natural background radiation. Ten gave me three quarters the cumulative radiation exposure as had been endured by the survivors of the Hiroshima atom bomb. The risk of a cancer from one barium meal I have seen quoted as one in a thousand; ten of them reduces the odds to one in a hundred, assuming there is no cumulative effect. However, it makes sense to me that there will be a cumulative effect so then the odds fall even further, not down to the level of a slam-dunk certainty, but surely a more likely cause than two weeks of Spanish sunshine thirty years prior.

Even when you see the same Crohn's medic for years on end as I had done to that point, it is difficult for them to step back and consider your lifetime's illness and treatment. Taken one at a time, my ten barium X-ray sessions each had benefits that outweighed the risks, but cumulatively I am not so sure. Would my Crohn's be any worse today if I had only had five?

Tip #77: You Have to Take Accountability for Your Medical Treatments

You have to take ownership for your treatment. Most times doctor does know best, but sometimes you have to use your own common sense and intuition. If it really doesn't feel right, push back and ask more questions. If still not happy, adopt the approach of the reluctant shopper and leave, saying you will "think about it" so you can do more research.

The next event is harder to pin directly on my Crohn's treatment, but there is enough of a smoking gun to convince me. At the time of my fifth operation, the one area of joy in what was a very tough time was that Audrey was five months pregnant with our first child. This had come as a complete shock to us both as we had, until about a year prior to the operation, been undergoing an increasingly invasive range of infertility treatments.

The first step in the process had been for me to undergo a sperm test. The deal was that I had to take a "sample" into the testing unit at our nearest hospital, and the "sample" could be no more than fifteen minutes old as they needed to observe the sperms' swimming techniques or something. So I had been sent off from the family doctor with a container and advice to get it to the clinic as early as possible the next day because the place was usually full once everyone had done the school run.

I immediately saw problems in carrying out these instructions. Firstly, even on a good run outside of rush hour, it took at least twenty minutes to drive from our house to the hospital, so getting the sample there within fifteen minutes was clearly going to be a problem. And secondly, I was not much of what might be termed a morning kind of guy. Thus, getting the sample there by 8.30 a.m., less than fifteen minutes old, still warm and full of gold medalist swimmers, was not going to be a simple matter of me retiring to the bathroom after downing the cornflakes and then taking a leisurely drive to the hospital.

We could think of no other solution than that the sample would have to be "produced" while parked up in the car at the hospital. Given the prospect of arrest and certain prosecution if some car park attendant spotted me alone on their premises conducting the exercise, Audrey was drafted in to provide a flimsy alibi that we could not keep our hands off each other and also devote all her skills to overcoming the tendency of my best friend to not reliably rise bright and early. I would then rush into the hospital with the container squashed into the crook of my armpit to keep it as warm as possible like a penguin sheltering its chick.

So, if you ever notice a car parked in the far distant corner of the hospital car park with the windows steamed up and creaking rhythmically on its suspension, you now know what's going on. It never ceases to amaze me just how little thought the medical profession puts into things like practicality and dignity.

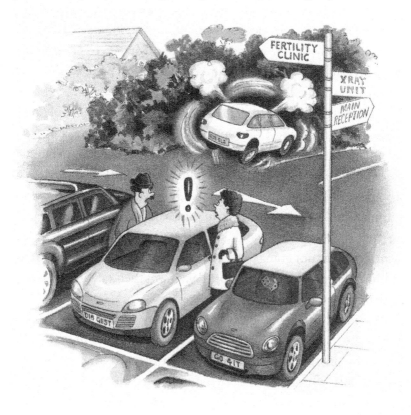

A handy place to park

Tip #78: You Have to Laugh

Find ways to laugh at the processes you are asked to endure, no matter how bizarre and inconvenient they may be. Otherwise you will explode with frustration.

When the test had been completed, it showed that all, on the face of it, seemed OK in the sperm department, so the focus naturally shifted to Audrey's egg production, even though she had become pregnant a couple of years into our marriage but had suffered a miscarriage. She was put on a fertility drug for six months whereby every four weeks or so her ovaries would feel like a midway popcorn machine going at full capacity. But it was to no avail as no pregnancy resulted so we were sent off to meet up with an infertility specialist which was an interesting affair.

We went as a couple and, for the first twenty-five minutes of our thirty-minute slot, I mutely played the role of the supportive husband while he quizzed Audrey, filling in several pages of a very long form. As his pen reached the very last box on this form, he turned to me.

"So Mr. Bradley, you are in good health I take it?"

"Errr, no, not really," I replied.

On hearing this, he raised his eyebrows, sighed, and reached into his desk for a completely different form. I got the impression he wished I had told him this upfront.

Tip #79: Don't Be Shy

In any new medical encounter, it's always a good idea to announce upfront that you have Crohn's disease. The advantages may not be immediately clear when one is at the, for example, Audiologist, but it's better to get into the habit with all of them.

After giving me an equally intense grilling on all my Crohn's treatments and operations, he opined that there probably wasn't a connection, but that one never knew. The next step would be another sperm test where they would be looking at other possible problems beyond sperm count. Being used to the arthritic pace of Ward 8, I naturally assumed that I would have to see the administrative assistant to get an appointment for a few weeks' time, but, much to my surprise and consternation, he reached into his drawer and took out a container.

"Room 2, second on the left."

Eeek! I wasn't ready for this, and what's more, we had visited during my work lunchtime and I was due back in fifteen minutes for a meeting. The pressure was on. Room 2 was a plush affair and came replete with quite a broad selection of top-shelfers, some of which looked suspiciously well-thumbed while others were pristine. It turned out on closer inspection that the untouched ones had clearly been bought by one of the more prudish staff members, being closer in style and content to RVing Weekly than Penthouse.

On our next visit, the gyno explained that, while I had a good sperm count, they were hamstrung by the fact that the seminal fluid contained antibodies to my own sperm. So, as soon as they were released, my body's immune system immediately set about killing them. It may have been that I had had this self-destruct mechanism for a long time and that, when Audrey had got pregnant, one sperm had survived the shock and awe and got through. (I preferred that explanation to the postman theory that Audrey jokingly put forward....) On the other hand, he explained, it could well be that, in one of my surgeries, something had been nicked and resulted in sperm getting into my bloodstream which would have then stimulated the production of antibodies which, as we all know from the fact we can only contract chicken pox once, never go away. It sounded pretty unlikely to me, but he darkly explained that all sorts of things happen in surgeries that are best not to know about.

But the good news was that they could "wash" the sperm immediately after production to remove the deadly antibodies before they could spring into action, and then inject the pristine sperm into Audrey's uterus, all within the usual fifteen minute deadline. So, on a monthly basis, I would rush down to the hospital during lunchtime, do my stuff, the sperm would go through the wash and spin cycle, get squirted up Audrey via the turkey baster, and then hopefully sperm would meet egg as if nothing untoward had happened. I would then rush back to work, go into the first afternoon meeting bright red in the face with beads of perspiration trickling down my forehead. This would invariably prompt questions along the lines of where I had been for my lunchtime run or had I been out for a particularly hot curry?

Alas, all this effort was in vain as no pregnancy resulted, so we then moved on to the last step before IVF, which was called GIFT – Gamete Intra-Fallopian Transfer where the eggs and sperm are mixed together then injected back into the fallopian tube but without having waited for conception to take place. This procedure cost an eye-watering $3,000, which was not covered by my insurance, and achieved nothing on our first attempt.

Tip #80: Know When to Draw the Line

It had been quite a traumatic process for Audrey, being a full anesthetic and keyhole surgery so, at this point, we ended our assisted conception efforts and resigned ourselves to being childless, almost certainly as a result of some surgical slip. Sometimes you have to call a halt when you feel the treatment is worse than the condition.

Interestingly, GIFT has almost disappeared from use today for two reasons. Firstly, its success rate has remained low while that of IVF has increased dramatically; and secondly, because it is so invasive. So it seems that we made a reasonable call. It's a good example of how sometimes you have to trust your own judgment against alleged medical science. Apparently, the only demand for it today comes from infertile, strict Catholics as the Pontiff has let this one through while he is still playing his veto card on IVF.

And, even better, there was a happy ending. As is often the case when couples give up trying, a few months later a miracle happened and we conceived naturally, a hardy and apparently invulnerable sperm successfully avoided the antibody storm troopers. Or perhaps Audrey's special postman really had rung twice....

After that happy ending, the next cross I had to bear resulting from my Crohn's and its treatments was the kidney stones that had been predicted by my fellow patients way back when. Not only had these old sages not exaggerated, in comparison to the actual event I endured, they had barely scratched the surface with their descriptions. If only kidney stones did feel like passing broken glass. I had no idea the body could produce such levels of pain. I had no warning that I even had kidney stones and within two minutes of wondering what that twinge was in my side as I was shaving one morning, I was so completely pole-axed with pain that Audrey called an ambulance.

Waiting for it to arrive and then the twenty-minute journey to the hospital was a complete nightmare, but then it seems the stone had made the excruciating journey from kidney to bladder by the time I was X-rayed as it was nestled at the bottom of my bladder. I have since read that kidney stones are as painful as childbirth. The same X-ray also showed a gallstone lurking in the gallbladder. This is still there, no doubt biding its time before crippling me at some inopportune moment. Both kidney and gallstones are conditions that can accompany Crohn's disease, especially when steroid treatment has been used.

Ironically, the treatment for dealing with steroid-induced bone loss is to take Vitamin D and calcium, both of which increase the chances of kidney stones. So would Sir prefer the rock, or, today's special, the hard place? The bone doctor tells me he would rather have kidney stones than osteoporosis, so I am following that advice even though he admitted he had never endured the unendurable pain of kidney stones. But he did know how bad osteoporosis can get so I took him at face value.

Tip #81: Rocks and Hard Places

You be the judge of what it is you want to suffer from. Don't let the doctor decide because then you will spend the rest of your life blaming him for picking the wrong one.

So after this depressing sequence of medical problems, it probably seems like things just go from bad to worse when you have Crohn's, which had been the case with me thus far. Although, by every measure, I was getting worse more quickly than ever before, much to my and the medics' surprise, the fifth operation for some unknown reason heralded a turning point in my fortunes.

Calmer Waters

"My doctor is nice; every time I see him, I'm ashamed of what I think of doctors in general."

— Mignon McLaughlin (American author 1913 – 1983)

MY FIFTH SURGERY had been the one with the least amount of time since the previous op, so I had little reason to think things would be getting better anytime soon. Being realistic, I would have been foolish to assume that this time all my troubles would be over. When I commenced negotiations with Cadbury as to my next posting, I made it clear that Cadbury World was not an option: The job was simply too taxing as a long-term prospect for me. But the turnaround had been a success so I could leave with my reputation intact if not enhanced. Even though I would be coming back feeling well, I was so concerned about how rapidly the last operation had come about that I decided it was time for another spell off the career escalator with a desk-bound job that would utilize my background and capabilities but not be too physically demanding with lots of travel or overly-long hours.

This desire fitted in with something my boss wanted to achieve in another part of his empire, so I was offered the role of head of commercial services, that being the area which contained various specialist departments such as market research, long range planning and the area where I had started my career and had already had two roles: market analysis and forecasting.

This was not necessarily a role that would have appealed to someone whose last two jobs had been in marketing and general manager of Cadbury World; many would have considered it a sideways move or even a backward step. Although the Cadbury World job had proved successful, I could not keep taking jobs that were as physically demanding and stressful as I would, at some stage, come spectacularly unstuck. If that ever happened, my career strategy would be down the tubes. So given how down I was about my prognosis, I was happy at that time to take on a role I knew to be well within my capability.

Tip #82: Keep Re-evaluating Your Career Strategy as Your Circumstances Change

Whether you are ill or not, past successes count for very little in the workplace. It is crucial that, even when you have managed to build a good reputation for yourself, you take nothing for granted. Heroes can become Zeroes if they are over-promoted or in the wrong job. You have to continue to make yourself invaluable to your employer. Once you start to use your health as an excuse for under-performance, it's only a matter of time before you lose control of your career, which can spell disaster.

You may have noticed by now a bit of a trend where my prolonged post-operative convalescences sometimes coincided with a switch in jobs. This was deliberate and, I believe, worked to the advantage of both Cadbury and myself. The benefit to me was that I was not leaving a hole that would create massive problems for the company, which would in effect be a switching of the burden of my health from my shoulders onto theirs. For their part, there was some element of being able to plan for both roles such that things went smoothly for everyone. So I returned to work in June 1993 after another fourteen-week layoff only to be back at home four weeks later on paternity leave following the birth of our beautiful daughter, Georgina. Since I was feeling well at this point, I was well able to withstand the sleepless nights.

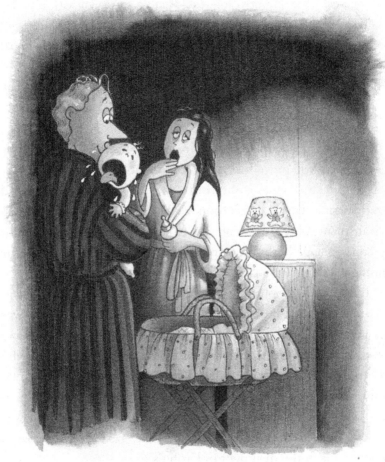

Bringing up Baby

Back at Cadbury, my caution about what kind of job to apply for proved to be wise. This time it was to be only six months before I was back in the Ward 8 clinic complaining that my symptoms were, once again, on the rise. Diarrhea, abdominal pain, no appetite, weight loss and more trouble with the rear end were all back as though they had never been away. After a couple of months of optimistically "seeing how it goes", I had a sit-down with Dr. Ray where we made some big decisions. Firstly, we agreed that there was no point doing another barium meal as we both knew what it would show – more strictures – so why add to my already cosmic levels of radiation? I was already glowing more at night than my watch dial.

The second decision was to restart the steroids but this time in conjunction with other drugs. There had been progress made since I last took steroids with some new research showing they could be more effective in preventing stricture formation if used in conjunction with a drug new to the treatment of Crohn's disease called Azathioprine. This had first been used by one of the great pioneers in transplant surgery to reduce the risk of organ rejection. It did so by suppressing the bone marrow and thus also suppressing the immune system response.

It had been adopted for use in Crohn's as, by this stage, it was becoming increasingly clear to researchers that Crohn's disease was an over-reaction of the body's immune system, perhaps in response to unknown bacteria in the gut that would not bother people who did not have this immune system flaw. There is some family trend in the incidence of Crohn's disease that pointed to a genetic mutation, although I had no relatives similarly afflicted. Thus, it was argued, drugs that inhibited the immune system could play a positive role in the treatment of Crohn's.

In this instance, I was more than ready to sign up for a new cocktail of drugs. The strategy over the past few years of not having any significant treatment would only lead, if continued, to more and more frequent visits to the operating theatre such that I doubted whether I would still be alive by the age of 40.

Tip #83: Balance the Risk of New Treatments Against the Benefits that Sometimes Come from the March of Science

If you feel you have no other choices, then sometimes you have to take a risk with new treatments. Having Crohn's is about balancing the three choices of feeling ill, undergoing surgery and being treated with drugs. Sometimes that balance will be changed by developments in one of the areas. There is no definitive "best option"; you just have to go with what looks like the least bad option at any point in time.

Of course, when contemplating new drugs, you have to do your homework. This time, I did not go to Birmingham's Central Library to learn all these facts, but had been informed by leaflets supplied by a Crohn's disease patients' charitable organization called the National Association for Crohn's and Colitis (NACC). Ulcerative Colitis being a condition somewhat similar to Crohn's, the two were invariably treated by the same specialists. This fine body had been formed by the parent of a Crohn's sufferer in the late 1970s to fill the then-gaping void of information for patients about their condition and to raise money to fund research into finding a cure. I had first come across NACC a couple of years after my diagnosis when a local branch of NACC was being set up with the Ward 8 clinic as its core member body.

It was at the NACC information meetings that I first became aware that my approach to having the illness was not one shared by the majority of sufferers. The surgeon who was to do my first four operations gave a marvelously entertaining and informative talk on the various surgical treatments for both Crohn's and Colitis. I kicked off with a question where I felt the answer would be of interest to the most members, asking what new surgical developments were in the pipeline. But after me came a host of audience members whose questions were solely about the peculiarities of either their symptoms or their treatment. In short, they were looking for a second opinion. Every meeting I have been to since that day has been exactly the same. It is not to say that I derived no benefit from NACC. I still find attending lectures to be a very useful source of knowledge and also encouragement that research is marching ever onwards towards better treatments and hopefully an eventual cure.

So what were the other differences that struck me so forcefully between my attitude to illness and that of others? As I mentioned at the start of this book, in my experience, 95% of fellow sufferers are either in complete denial or, to varying degrees, consider their lives to have been ruined, or at least to be somewhat substandard, compared to either what they were expecting for themselves or to how they perceived the lives of "normal" people. Almost by definition, the deniers were not likely to become members of an organization like NACC, thus leaving the vast majority of members as people who were looking primarily for personal support, comfort or a shoulder to cry on. There is nothing wrong with that as long as the patient doesn't allow it to degenerate into a "woe is me" approach to life, which, while understandable, is never helpful.

I think I can best summaries my outlook on my illness as follows. Firstly, in life we have to play the hand we are dealt. Yes, being ill is not pleasant and it would be better to not be ill, but if life was fair, we would all be living in a Mumbai or Lagos slum with nothing to eat tonight. Secondly, I see my disease as not a depressing burden that hampers my life's progress, but as a life-partner from an arranged marriage to whom I have to make certain concessions compared to what I would do if I did not have it. I did not choose this partner and I cannot get rid of it, so why let these unchangeable circumstances potentially ruin my life? Thirdly, there are many other aspects of my life where I feel exceptionally blessed and one must always try to look at the bigger picture. I still feel that, even with the course my Crohn's has taken, 97% of the world's population would gladly switch places with me, so what am I complaining about?

Tip #84: Above All Else, Stay Positive

Most of the tips I have passed on from my journey of learning are practical ones on how best to deal with doctors, hospitals, symptoms and career planning. But these are not enough. I offer you the central thought that you have to keep the positive mindset that the rest of your life can still be incredibly rich and fulfilling, just different to the one you thought you were going to have.

Much to my amazement, not only did I feel better by being on the steroids/Azathioprine mix, but my Crohn's symptoms gradually receded, culminating in the second butt hole healing itself! I was still not able to completely get off the steroids without the symptoms returning, but was able to keep myself feeling good enough off a much lower dose than had been the case years previously. My maintenance dosage was 10mg/day which compares to the body's usual production rate of its own natural steroids of 7mg/day. In the past I couldn't get below 25mg/day.

This meant that I had very few obvious steroid-related symptoms to bother me but I did have the illusion of feeling well that came from a slightly elevated dosage. Thus, the next two years were very calm waters as far as my health was concerned. I was aware there were one or two strictures in my system, but, if I continued to be vigilant in chewing my food to a mush and avoiding mushrooms, sweet corn and peanuts completely, I suffered no ill effects. My visits to the Ward 8 clinic (by now transplanted into another hospital) became less frequent as there was no new news to report. The first time I was given an appointment for six months' time I did a jig of delight walking back down the corridor as I had never had one of these before in the past dozen years. It was the appointment slot given to patients who were stable whereas I was always, "Come back in four weeks, Mr. Bradley." Finally!

I gradually got used to feeling well and expecting to feel well. I could make social appointments and know I would keep them. We could accept dinner invitations safe in the knowledge I would clear my plate. I am to this day amazed at how everyone else seems to take completely for granted the wonderful sensations of feeling hungry, eating a big meal, and feeling replete afterwards. It is far better than sex and, what's more, you can enjoy it three times a day, every day without attracting undue attention or collapsing through exhaustion.

Feeling well for a prolonged period had certainly been a long time coming. It had been at least fifteen years since I had been similarly untroubled. I tried not to over-analyze the turnaround or shout too loudly from the rooftops as it could all have ended the next day. Probably the main change mentally was that I was conscious of gradually thinking less and less about my health which meant that I got increasing amounts of enjoyment from even the most mundane of daily activities.

The only downside to my recovery was that, as time went by, I began to get bored in my job so started looking for the next career escalator to climb on. Probably spurred on a bit by the steroids, when looking around Cadbury for another job, I became interested in the idea of taking a placement in one of Cadbury's overseas divisions. Of course, even though I was feeling well, I could not go into this process blindly as I might not be feeling well at some point in the future, so I had to be very careful as to the countries I considered for such a move.

So I decided that I had to be much more open with the company about my health/career planning strategy than I had been to date. Until this point, I had kept my strategy largely to myself; I thought the less my employer ever thought about my health, the better. But now I had to confess as there was no possibility, because of my health, that I would ever sign up for a move to, for example, Cadbury Nigeria or Cadbury Indonesia, and blank refusal of such roles might have been misinterpreted. So I approached the person in the global head office who was responsible for facilitating overseas moves and came clean as to my thinking.

To my mind, the benefit of having people looking out for roles based on my health requirements might have been outweighed by being tagged a "special case" in too many minds. My goal had always been to make my performance and delivery of results well worth any inconvenience brought about by me having time off. I did not want to add any further inconveniences, which is how I saw having people thinking about what was best for me as opposed to what was best for the company, even when it was their job to do so. I never used my health as an excuse for under-performance so I didn't want to use it as an excuse for any special treatment. But, in this case, I had to.

Tip #85: Consciously Decide How Much to Share With Your Employer

How much you share with your employer depends on what kind of employer they are and how comfortable you are sharing such things. I have never been much of a sharer and am happy to accept that I may be off towards one end of the spectrum. What you must do, however, is what feels right for you.

The bottom line in our discussion on possible locations was that I could only consider a move to a country that had a top-notch health system that was free to use. I could not consider going to countries where any difficult or emergency health problem could not be treated expertly there and then. I could also not consider going to America where health care is insurer funded and at that time would most definitely have excluded me as being a walking textbook of pre-existing conditions.

I have been asked many times about health insurance for my Crohn's; the assumption being from most questioners that it is an option. I have to inform them that it is not. Health insurers are not in the business of spending large sums of money paying for the care of sick people; they are in the business of taking money off healthy people or their employers. I have never seen a health insurance option that does not specifically exclude Crohn's and all its many symptoms as a pre-existing condition.

Tip #86: Health Insurance is for the Healthy

Take out life insurance and private medical insurance before you become ill, because no one will cover you when you face a lifetime of medical interventions.

When we looked at an atlas and stuck pins in the countries that met my health criteria and also had a Cadbury subsidiary, there were four: Ireland, Australia, New Zealand and Canada, so it was a case of waiting for suitable vacancies to arise in one of those locations. A month after my meeting, head office called to say that a vacancy in the Canadian business had indeed arisen. At first I was not too interested. Even in the context of my career escalator strategy, this looked not like heading up to the next floor but going back down to menswear. The job was definitely smaller than the one I had and in a much smaller business unit. So I said, "No thanks."

But I then had a word with the senior executive in charge of all Cadbury's operations in the Americas, who had recently taken several managers over there from other countries. He had previously worked for many years in Cadbury's UK marketing department, so he was well aware of the health problems I had endured. His advice was that moving country was an extremely stressful experience so, if I was only going to move for a promotion into a bigger job, it would be piling stress level upon stress level. My health might be good now, but was it wise to subject it to what would have been its ultimate challenge to date? After considering it, Audrey and I decided that this was good advice, so I asked that my name be put forward.

This was a good example of how, when your health recovers and symptoms become dim and distant memories – a process that happens surprisingly rapidly – it is easy to slip into the mindset that you are not ill at all. It is hard to hold yourself back when you are feeling well, but I believe it is important to at least consider doing so. Illness, surgery and drug regimes do take a toll, so it is foolish to think that you have suddenly become indestructible. You always need something in the tank for when things go wrong, as they inevitably will with chronic conditions. If I had held out for a promotion on an overseas assignment, and my health had suffered accordingly, it would have been putting the problem in the company's lap to repatriate us and find me another job at relatively short notice.

Tip #87: Remember You Are Still Ill When You Feel Well

While I am an advocate of enjoying the moment, there is no point just creating problems for yourself down the line by being too ambitious in your plans when you are feeling well. The hard bit is to not let that process get out of hand and you end up never achieving anything.

We were invited over to Toronto for a week in August 1996 for me to be interviewed. This went well as, a week after we got back to England, I was offered the job on the basis of a two-year assignment. On November 10, 1996, we bid farewell to our sobbing parents at Birmingham airport and headed off to our new life.

Moving country is indeed a stressful exercise. You are overwhelmed with information and you can do nothing on automatic pilot as everything is different to a greater or lesser extent. But once we had ploughed through the house move and finding our feet, a big focus for me was to meet up with the healthcare infrastructure that had been lined up by Cadbury's company medic, these being a local family doctor in the town where we had decided to live and also a Crohn's disease specialist at one of Toronto's main teaching hospitals.

It was apparent on first meetings with both these doctors that things worked a little bit differently in Canada compared to back in England. This being North America, where convenience is a way of life, the family doctor's office, along with those of a couple of dozen other family doctors, was part of a health practice that also included X-ray and ultrasound facilities, a blood test clinic, an after-hours walk-in clinic and a pharmacy. One-stop shopping for anything but the most serious of health needs.

Our new family doctor, who was a genial Welshman nearing retirement age, was able to explain other differences between the Canadian and British systems. Medical care was free in both countries, being funded out of taxation. In Canada though, prescriptions were neither free nor subsidized but were covered by employers as part of employee wellness plans. More interestingly, he explained what he considered to be key attitudinal differences. The family doctors in Canada took more ownership for the total healthcare of the patient. They would visit you in hospital and, if you were not happy with a specialist, they could transfer you to another one merely by sending a letter asking the new one to take you on. Equally, my doctor predicted that I would find the specialists to be much less aloof and God-like in their attitude to patients than had been the case in the UK.

I soon found this to be the case when I went to meet the gastroenterologist. He was an extremely friendly guy who seemed bowled over that he had inherited a patient from the now defunct Birmingham Royal Free Hospital, which apparently was world famous in the Crohn's medical community. He had heard of both Dr. Ray and my surgeon. He also took great pains in telling me that things worked slightly differently in Canada. He didn't see hundreds of patients at a time aided by cohorts of juniors in formal clinics. Every time I saw him it would be one-on-one in his office. If anything changed or I needed something I just had to call and leave a message. More often than not, he would call back that same evening, discuss whatever was on my mind and even arrange new or repeat prescriptions with a phone call to my local pharmacy. Quite a change.

Since I had the opportunity of a clean sheet in terms of my relationships with these doctors, and things seemed a little more flexible in terms of how people worked, I set out to execute a strategy in my dealings with doctors that had been formulating in my mind for quite a while. This was that I should see each different kind of doctor in a different light, rather than view them as one largely homogenous mass, which I believe most patients do. If I could leverage the differences between the doctors by how I dealt with them, I could perhaps end up with a better standard of healthcare than the average.

Tip #88: Make the Family Doctor the Centre of Your Healthcare Strategy

Most patients who also see a specialist tend to cut the family doctor out of the equation on the grounds that they are not experts in the specific condition; their knowledge invariably being sketchy, out-of-date, and clearly inferior to that possessed by the specialist. All of this may be true but, to my mind, is largely irrelevant. The family doctor is not meant to be a substitute for the specialist and he/she should be your best friend in the medical system – I guarantee it will pay dividends.

My reasoning behind this goes as follows. Because many chronically ill patients bypass the family doctor, the poor medic is left dealing with the malingerers, hypochondriacs and the aged – hardly what they dreamt about during all those years studying. However, if I did the opposite to the herd and fully involved the family doctor in everything, they would so enjoy dealing with a real patient who had a real illness that they would be motivated to go above and beyond on my behalf.

What, you may ask, does "above and beyond" mean if they don't know much about Crohn's disease? Quite a lot actually.

Where they are far more expert than the specialists is in the overall workings of the health system. Being located in the community, they have an outsider's perspective on the hospital-based system but far more knowledge than you and I on how it works. They are also, I have found, far more responsive and proficient in dealing with the side-effects of your treatments and surgeries as they treat you, the entire patient, not just some obscure condition.

Our Welsh family doctor retired a few years ago and was replaced by a younger, female doctor who had previously been a nurse and had then retrained. I see her several times a year, not to complain or treat her like a doormat, but to seek her advice. I send her a personalized Christmas card every year and take a gift for her office staff (relationships you should also invest time and effort in). She is my perfect medical partner: her nursing background means she is well aware of the many drawbacks of doctors, specialists and hospitals. I really do believe that I am not just a patient number to her but that she has my interests at heart.

Tip #89: Measure Your Doctor Against the Standards Set by Their Patron Saint, Hippocrates:

"(He) routinely tasted his patients' urine, sampled their pus and earwax, and smelled and scrutinized their stool. He assessed the stickiness of their sweat and examined their blood, their phlegm, their tears, and their vomit. He became closely acquainted with their general disposition, family and home, and he studied their facial expressions. In deciding upon a final diagnosis and treatment, Hippocrates recorded and considered dietary habits, the season, the local prevailing winds, the water supply at the patient's residence, and the direction the home faced."[i]

Now that's what I call a doctor! It's a pity that the Hippocratic Oath doesn't include all this as being mandatory practice. Although my family doctor doesn't quite go this far, she invariably takes my side and helps me strategies against the biggest enemy the medical world can throw at you – the specialist.

The next time you are confronted by a specialist who talks to you as though you are a simpleton, conveys the impression that the course of your illness is fully understood, that all treatments will work and the best thing you can do is keep your opinions to yourself, it's time to take your business elsewhere. Like most people, I started my medical journey assuming, based largely on television dramas, that the specialist is the hero, but I am now very wary of them. They are prone to mistake knowledge for wisdom. The Doctor = God syndrome is most pronounced in the specialist community, so they can be the most difficult of the medics to deal with.

Tip #90: Keep Shopping Around for Your Specialist

Be quick to take your business elsewhere if you are not happy with your specialist. I am now on my third gastroenterologist in Canada for reasons that will become clear in the next chapter.

---

[i] David H. Newman, *Hippocrates' Shadow*, (Scribner, New York, 2008), pp xiii-xiv

The surgeon is a different matter entirely. You must not judge them by normal criteria. A bit like the fact that all good insurance sales people are nightmares to be stuck with in an enclosed space, all good surgeons are completely overbearing. If, when you meet a surgeon, you don't come out feeling like you have been hit by a human hurricane, look for another. Knowledge, experience, confidence and expertise are everything. Despite what the anatomy manuals say, no two bodies are the same inside, so you want a surgeon who has seen it all. The best surgeons tend to work in the best hospitals and use the best theatre staff and anesthetists – they don't want their batting averages ruined by having surrounded themselves with incompetents. So try to avoid the hacker at a local hospital for all but the most basic procedures. You also need to beware of surgeons who seem determined to build a reputation for themselves as that can lead to a tendency to push the envelope a little too far.

Tip #91: Ask Your Family Doctor – Would You Let This Surgeon Operate on Your Child?

A well-established family doctor will know which surgeon is the washed-up slasher, which is the over-aggressive risk-taker and which they would trust with their loved one's life. Make sure to get an honest opinion about a surgeon before you agree to be sliced open.

Although I had been feeling well enough for long enough to feel confident in making the move to Canada, it did not mean that I was illness-free – chronic conditions by definition never go away – nor was I entirely symptom-free. I was still prone to the various complications of the disease itself and also those flowing from having had five major surgeries, each one of which had shortened my small bowel. In fact, as time went by, I came to the conclusion that most of my niggling symptoms resulted from the cumulative surgeries rather than from new manifestations of the illness itself.

After frequent and invasive contact with the medical profession over a twenty-year time period, you will without question face two health problems: that of the illness itself and that resulting from your treatment. You may feel that you are worse off than ever before because the effects from the treatment tend to accumulate over time. This is the real price you pay for getting ill in the first place. But, because they accumulate slowly over time, you just assimilate each one into the normality of your life and move on. I have avoided mushrooms for so long now, I never even think of having one, let alone drool at the thought.

Tip #92: Keep Looking Forward

As the manifestations of your treatment begin to accumulate, constantly looking back to the halcyon days before you were ill and comparing your life now to your life then is not a good idea. You need to be always looking forward when afflicted with Crohn's. Looking forward to plan how you can avoid many of the pitfalls I have described in this book, and also looking forward to the days when you feel somewhat better.

By and large, the changes brought about by my cumulative treatments were inconvenient rather than debilitating. At some stage during my early years in Canada I developed lactose intolerance. This comes about when your body produces insufficient quantities of the enzyme lactase, which acts to break down the indigestible complex sugar lactose into simple sugars that can be easily absorbed by the gut. It seemed that the portion of my digestive system responsible for producing lactase had either been chopped out or become diseased.

The lactose issue did raise in my consciousness whether or not I should take more seriously the role of diet in the management of my condition. I already knew that drinking the gallons of elemental diet every day and resting the bowel from most regular foods did in fact reduce the symptoms of active inflammation. Also, in much of the NACC literature, there were many examples of where people cutting out wheat or even all carbohydrate had made some improvement, though I must confess that I have always shied away from such draconian measures as a way of life. I went for so long not enjoying a single morsel that I simply could not face the thought of voluntarily denying myself the pleasures of a regular diet.

Tip #93: Don't Give Up All Your Pleasures

Sometimes one has to trade off the discomfort of the symptoms for the pleasure of the indulgence. Of course, it is up to you how you approach trade-offs such as these, but I have found that you need the occasional pleasures to keep your spirits up, even if they come with a big price tag in the bathroom.

The next medical event was a recurrence of the dreaded kidney stones. This time, I was stricken in the middle of a meeting at work. If anything, the time taken from onset of the first twinge to me writhing on the floor chewing on the carpet was even faster than the first time – I estimate about 2.3 seconds. Knowing what it was, I was able, gasping between spasms, to calm the fears of the other members of the Marketing Appropriations Committee who had swiftly moved from thinking how badly I was taking the decision to reduce my PR budget to being horrified at what looked like a life-threatening emergency.

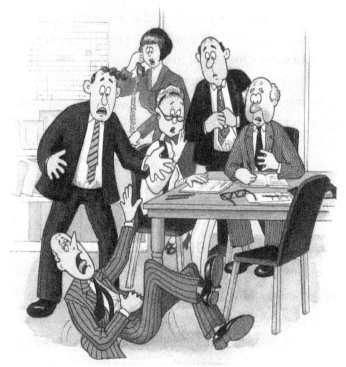

A painful meeting

Unlike the previous occurrence when the pain had disappeared within the space of a couple of minutes, this time it only gradually abated. I went to the walk-in clinic (crawl-in would be a better description of how I entered it) at my family doctor's where an X-ray showed that the stone appeared to be stuck half-way along the urethra, the tube between my left kidney and the bladder. The solution to this dilemma was a quick referral to a kidney specialist at a Toronto teaching hospital who then equally quickly arranged for me to have a technique known in the kidney trade as Extracorporeal Shock Wave Lithotripsy where the stone was to be blasted to smithereens by sound waves. I thought the whole procedure to be a marvelous use of science and technology.

Technology had also been on the march in the treatment of Crohn's disease, which I was to benefit from a year or two after the kidney stone pulverizing. Once again, it seems I had been insidiously bleeding from somewhere in my small bowel and become grossly anemic. Just like last time, I did not figure out for myself that I had become anemic, but it depended on a chance comment from a colleague from my Cadbury UK days who I met up with on a course. They knew me well enough to feel comfortable pointing out that, in their view, I looked very pale. Neither Audrey nor I had noticed the gradual decline as we were too close to see the wood for the trees.

Tip #94: Never Neglect Your Wellness Radar

I find that you have to encourage people to speak their minds when they think things might not be going well with your health. Most will keep their concerns to themselves assuming either that a) you already know, or b) they don't want to worry you. Constantly encourage your relatives, close friends and colleagues to speak up if they see a change in you.

A blood test showed that I was indeed anemic to the point that iron tablets would not restore my rosy complexion on their own, so a round of blood transfusions was required. This one went smoothly but I was back again a month later as I seemed to have bled it all out again without my knowing it. My gastroenterologist hypothesized that, while I obviously had a bit of bleeding somewhere in the small bowel, perhaps the bigger problem was my body not making up the loss as fully as it should. This could be due to a deficiency of Vitamin B12 which is necessary to help the body convert iron from tablets (of which I was by now taking a regular dose) into hemoglobin. As B12 was produced naturally by the end portion of the small bowel, which I had long since lost to surgery, it seemed my body's stores had finally run out. So I was put on monthly injections of B12, which will be an omnipresent feature for the rest of my life, and that seemed to succeed.

Despite this successful intervention, I had become increasingly concerned that I might be better off if I was seeing a different gastroenterologist. The one who had taken my case when we first arrived in Canada had decided that the irritants I was suffering might be caused by my small bowel being a little too short to cope rather than by a recurrence of inflammation. This was a plausible theory – after five surgeries, my bowel was well under half its normal length – but it did not sit well with me as it precluded him from considering other treatments for Crohn's than the steroid plus immunosuppressant regime I had been on for nearly a decade.

I went to discuss the issue with my family doctor, who, it transpired, had also been having reservations herself as she had not been kept as fully in the loop about my phone calls and visits with the gastroenterologist as she would have liked. As chance would have it, the next week was one of the bi-annual lecture meetings of our local branch of the Canadian equivalent of NACC, called the Crohn's and Colitis Foundation of Canada. The keynote speaker was the head of the gastroenterology department at a University teaching hospital. Both Audrey and I were very impressed with the speaker, so asked our family doctor to arrange for me to be transferred to be under her care. I had done my research on her which included getting a recommendation from my old gastroenterologist in the UK, to whom I had written asking if he knew of any top gastroenterologists in Canada. The transfer process happened seamlessly and my first meeting with her confirmed in my mind that I had been right to move. I liked this consumer-centric approach to healthcare where the patient was boss.

Laugh? I Nearly Died!

"Until the physician has killed one or two, he is not a physician."

— **Kashmiri Proverb**

AFTER MY INITIAL consultation with the new gastroenterologist, her take on the situation was that she believed I was not suffering from short bowel syndrome but that the Crohn's was once again active. This meant the steroid therapy was not working; a problem compounded by the fact that she was of the opinion I had become steroid dependent, which was not a good thing given the dire complications that can result from long-term steroid therapy.

Her suggestion was to wean me off the steroids – a process that would take months – and replace them in my care regimen with a new drug that had only recently been licensed for use in Canada, which operated on completely different principles. This drug had been mentioned by the previous guy, but he had shied away from putting me on it as it would have done nothing for a short bowel.

It is not a case of one doctor being right and one doctor being wrong. Medicine is much more an art based on opinion than a science based on fact, though you would not think so given the absolute certainty conveyed by every doctor in every pronouncement they make. So I felt good about having made the change of specialist because this new doctor's opinion made more sense to me and fitted better with my view of both what was wrong and what was the best way forward.

Tip #95: Doctors Will Always Disagree

Studies have shown that doctors not only readily disagree with the opinions of other doctors in things like the interpretation of electrocardiograms – up to 75% of the time – but also disagree with themselves if unknowingly presented with the same test results to review again. So you should expect some differences of opinion. That being the case, you are better off seeing a doctor with whom you have a shared perspective on your condition as opposed to one you are forever locking horns with.

The new drug, Infliximab, was and is a miracle of modern science. Genetically engineered in laboratory mice, it works by disrupting the chemical messengers in the bloodstream that are part of the inflammation process. Thus, it does not do anything to cure the illness, but prevents the inflammation in the small bowel that is the source of stricture formation. But, and there is always a but, there are some downsides. Firstly, it is fantastically expensive at $5,000 for each infusion, but fortunately, after a bit of negotiation, that was covered by my employer's drug plan. Secondly, as it was so new, little was known about side effects, particularly from long-term use. Thirdly, it was to be delivered via a drip into my vein once every eight weeks, a process that took half a day and had to be conducted in a specialized clinic with a doctor nearby in case of allergic reaction. And fourthly, once I had started taking the drug, I could not stop eating cheese (OK, I made that one up).

I was keen to try the new therapy but, being realistic, what choice did I have? Compared to the risks of continued steroid treatment and the certainty of more symptoms that would undoubtedly result in another surgery without any drug treatment, I felt I had little to lose and much to gain by opting for the new drug. As the new gastroenterologist pointed out to me, ten years was already far too long to have been on steroids. I had already had some fairly major negative effects and was putting myself at risk of ones that were much worse, such as diabetes, glaucoma and cataracts. In addition to avoiding these drastic problems, the other good news was that long-term steroid use could result in a reduced sex drive, so getting off them had the potential to turbo-charge my libido. This prompted in the Bradley household a few retellings of the good old joke about me needing to have sex six times a week and Audrey putting her name down for three of them.

Tip #96: Keep Up-to-Date on Developments

Don't get stuck in a rut of keeping with a past decision that has since been overtaken by events. New drugs are being invented all the time and genetic engineering has opened up many more avenues of potential treatment. Being able to keep up-to-date on new developments is one of the major benefits of becoming a member of a patient organization such as NACC or CCFC. It gives you the ammunition to quiz your specialist as to new treatment options.

New technology had also been on the march in the field of being able to see what was going on inside my bowel. Until this point, the only window on the course of my illness had been from the dreaded barium meals and enemas, which were now the last thing I wanted to endure given my tendency to send Homeland Security Geiger-counters at the airport into overdrive. My new gastroenterologist announced that she was able to borrow from the manufacturer a new and improved endoscope that could be pushed far down into the deeper recesses of the small bowel. The previous model had not been able to get much past the first bend beyond the stomach, so this was a major advance. Since she was still worried that we had never identified the causes of my recent blood loss, she was keen to road-test this miraculous machine on me and take the first real-time look-see into my small bowel.

As with a normal endoscopy, it was a day-surgery procedure that involved me being sedated but still vaguely awake. But this time I was not sedated enough for my liking as the first stage of the procedure felt exactly like someone trying to ram a garden hose down my throat. My response, not unnaturally, was to frantically claw at the thing and try and pull it out, which prompted the nurse to pin me down and the gastroenterologist to give a much heavier lean on the sedation plunger, sending me into a delayed but much welcomed oblivion.

On waking, I was fascinated to see the pictures she had taken in there, these being the first new images of my insides since Cheryl's snapshots over twenty years earlier. The gastroenterologist explained that she had been able to push the scope about six or seven feet into my system until her way was blocked by a stricture. This had narrowed the bowel down to a gap of about 1/6th of an inch wide compared to the usual half inch or more. Even though she had not been able to push past, by snuggling the camera and light right up to the opening, she had been able to peek through and see another, similar stricture further on down. Both looked like they had been there quite some time, most probably having formed in the first six months after my last operation that was by then nearly a decade ago.

The good news was that it seemed no new strictures had formed; the bad news being that these old ones would have to be removed sooner or later. Since my symptoms at this stage were more annoying and inconvenient than debilitating, I voted for later, especially as the new drug had the potential to prevent further stricture formation without the potentially cataclysmic damage that steroids could do to my health. Thus, we transitioned to the new drug regime and all seemed well.

Perhaps perversely at this stage, since I was as well and stable as I had been in my adult life, I took the decision to finally exit the corporate world and leave Cadbury. By now I was forty-six years old and had come to the realization that continuing to pursue the career path I was on would be a mistake. The demands of the level I was at, having been promoted twice while in the Canadian business, seemed to just keep going up and up. This was not an issue unique to Cadbury but was one I could see happening to executives everywhere. Hours were getting longer; e-mail and BlackBerries meant that you were always on-call. I felt I had reached the stage where I could no longer balance success in this kind of career with putting my health first, and I wanted to get out before I had to compromise either one.

Tip #97: Quit While You Are Still Ahead

It is crucial to know when to get out. There might well come a point where any more success at work could take you into a position where you will probably fail at both the job and managing your health. Even robustly healthy people burn out, so do not leave it too late to consider other options.

So on October 31, 2003, I left the only company I had ever worked for to set myself up as a self-employed marketing consultant, giving myself four years to earn a living before I would be able to take an early retirement pension at the age of fifty. While being self-employed might sound even more stressful, I had a generous severance package and we also took the further precaution of downsizing our house to pay off the mortgage. Thus, I did not need to go out working every available hour, but could work at a gentler pace.

This turned out to be a wise move in many ways. Working from home left me feeling much better than when I had been toiling away on the corporate treadmill. I hadn't realized just how exhausted I had felt in the evenings while working full-time, nor how much more relaxed I would feel during the day without the endless meetings. Career-induced stress is insidious in that, because it is there all the time, you think it normal, not even realizing that you are feeling stressed.

Although I had always rejected stress as a primary cause of my illness and its symptoms, there is no doubt that stress makes you feel worse when you already have something. So permanent, low-level stress coupled with a chronic condition was always going to have left me feeling less than ideal. But I had no choice up to the point when I left Cadbury; I had had to build a career during the prolonged period of ill-health and multiple surgeries if I was to have any kind of reasonable life.

The four years following my departure from the workplace were the best run I had ever had in terms of feeling well. Of course I still had the irritating effects of the strictures, but the Infliximab seemed to be keeping any new ones at bay and the prospect of full-scale open surgery seemed a steam hammer to crack a nut, so I never even considered it. From having five surgeries in ten years, it had by this point been over ten years without one. I could never have predicted such a run and our move to Canada had definitely been the right one as I had been able to fast-track my career while my illness was at bay.

Things then changed when I met with a surgeon at the hospital who was developing a keyhole surgery approach to dealing with strictures. On the face of it, this seemed a terrific idea but, after my discussion with him, I was less than keen. I had had so much surgery in the past that I was extremely nervous about undergoing what always seemed to me a less than precise surgical technique. My insides would by now look nothing like anyone else's, so I was less than convinced that he would be able to easily navigate his way around. Even the surgeon seemed dubious (which was a first in my experience), giving his opinion that if we went ahead there would be an 80% chance he would have to abandon the approach halfway through and open me up to do the job in the traditional way. I decided to wait until technology had advanced some more.

In September 2007, I was sent off to see another specialist member of the staff, this time someone who had adopted a new technology recently invented in Japan called a Double Balloon Enteroscopy. This devilishly cunning piece of kit combined the extra-long enteroscope that had plumbed the depths of my bowel a couple of years before with the balloon idea that is used to open up narrowed arteries from within, in this case being used to widen strictures. When I quizzed the man on how many he had done, his reply was a somewhat reassuring seventy-ish. Since I had been the third recipient of a strictureplasty, this seemed a well-established practice by comparison and perhaps was another such new technique that could transform my prospects.

Of course I went on the internet to look up this technology and found a video made by the inventor himself showing the inside story of a stricture being torn to shreds. There was a bit of internal bleeding but nothing too drastic. The only stated downside was a small chance, circa 4%, of the equipment perforating the bowel wall which would then require immediate emergency surgery. This was a sobering thought but, on the positive side, here was exactly the kind of medical advance I had been waiting for all these years. Strictures had always been the main manifestation of my illness, but the resolution of them through open surgery was both traumatic and very debilitating.

When I went back to see the man, my mind was almost made up to volunteer for it, but what sealed the deal was the news that, in a couple of weeks' time, the pioneer of the technique in North America would be at this very hospital to demonstrate it at a gastroenterology conference. They were looking for suitable patients to undergo the procedure that would be beamed on closed-circuit television to a nearby hotel where three hundred gastroenterologists would be watching it on the big screen.

I thought this was a great idea. I would be getting the most ex-perienced practitioner of the technique in the entire continent who would surely be on top of his game given he was showing off to three hundred of his industry peers. So I eagerly agreed, with the proviso that I wanted to have a full anesthetic – I didn't want the same awareness of the tube going down that I had suffered the last time – plus an overnight stop just to make sure there had been no perforation.

Two weeks later I was back in the hospital, having starved for two days, ready and waiting for my turn on the big screen. I met the hot-shot just minutes before being wheeled into the room and given my anesthetic, so had little chance to size him up personally. When I groggily came round, I was in the recovery ward along with a few other equally adventurous patients who had been on show after me. I was told I would be kept there for a few hours just to make sure all was well, but, a few hours later, it was becoming increasingly clear from the number of worried-looking medics who came to check my vitals, that all was not well. Eventually, the mobile X-ray unit was called to image my abdomen which showed that my small bowel had indeed been perforated.

I would be lying if I said I took this news in my stride – it was a major disappointment and I was by no means looking forward to undergoing open surgery number six. But, I kept telling myself, it was a risk that had been worth taking. As I waited for a surgeon to be rustled up, I could not help pondering why this perforation of my bowel had not been apparent during the procedure itself. The 'scope had a camera on the front end and there were three hundred specialized gastroenterologists staring at the live footage. Surely one of them might have noticed the scope poking through the bowel wall like the monster that had burst out of John Hurt's stomach in Alien? But apparently not, or the medical code of omertà was even stronger than I had previously thought.

I must admit to now being extremely dubious when I hear statistics on how often complications occur. They are always small percentages and are told in a way that you get the impression it is always a random event. Since the odds are always on your side, why wouldn't you always sign up? I now believe when they say such and such a complication occurs 4% of the time, it does not mean that each of us has a 4% chance of something going wrong. What it really means is there are 4% of patients for whom it is almost certain to happen, and 96% for whom it will never happen.

In hindsight, the amount of surgery I had undergone in the past meant that, with so many surgically-inflicted loops and sharp bends, I was in the doomed 4%. If I had realized this at the time, I would never have signed up; my symptoms were not worth undergoing a full, open surgery.

Tip #98: Think Long and Hard About the Risks

When you have a procedure coming up, be sure to ask what the main complications are and how commonly they occur. Ask what factors seem to affect the risk level. Then follow up with detailed questions about there being any features of your case that would increase any of those risks. If they can't answer the questions immediately and knowledgeably, you need to be very wary indeed.

Before being taken down for surgery, I was wheeled to the main ward to stake my claim on a bed. The doctor in charge told me that he had telephoned Audrey, who was on her way in, but, before she arrived, the news came through that they were ready for me in theatre, so I was then wheeled out towards the elevators. On my way there, I saw two adults and a teenager in the distance, this turning out to be Audrey and Georgina along with a family friend, Gregg, who had kindly driven them into Toronto. By now it was eight o'clock at night, so I suggested to Audrey they would be better off going back home as, by the time I came out, it would be late at night and I didn't want to be worrying about them.

So we then parted as we had done five times previously (although first time for Georgina), each to our own private thoughts as I was wheeled to theatre. Personally, my predominant emotion was being annoyed with myself for having become an emergency, which was something I had always tried to avoid. While I was very apprehensive about the rigors of surgery and the prolonged recuperation, having undergone this five times before, I was not unduly worried. But I should have been.

I remember very little of what happened in the aftermath of the surgery, although things seemed to be on track. Audrey received a phone call at around 10:30pm from the surgeon saying that all had gone well and I was being taken back up to the ward. Early the next morning, Audrey called the ward to see how I had slept during the night and was immediately put on her guard by what she thought was an evasive response, along the lines of there being no one who could come to the phone right now as things were rather busy.

What she wasn't told was that things were rather busy because my room was full of doctors frantically trying to get blood and fluids into my veins. During the night I had suffered a catastrophic internal hemorrhage and had gone into an almost fatal hypovolemic shock, this being where the blood loss is so great that the heart just does not have enough fluid to pump round the system. I myself was dimly aware of some major drama going on when hands grabbed my neck, groin and ankle in attempts to detect what was by then a very faint pulse. I was also vaguely aware of drips being inserted into both my arms to try and get as much volume of blood and fluid back into my system, and I remember hearing a doctor shouting, "Open it up full," which was referring to setting the drips to run at full bore. I discovered later that the amount of blood plasma and fluids being pumped into me constituted an exceptionally aggressive and risky procedure that was essentially kill or cure and could easily have gone horribly wrong. But I was literally at death's door because of the huge volume of blood I had already lost.

While this pandemonium was going on, an operating theatre was being readied and I was rushed down for my second emergency surgery within the space of twelve hours. All the blood and fluids forced into my system had temporarily restored me to a semi-consciousness and I was certain in my mind that I was going to die. They didn't even bother holding me up in the pre-op room as I was taken straight into the theatre. Somewhat bizarrely, I was asked to sign a consent form at this point, the surgeon basically summarizing that they had no idea what had gone wrong inside and that I should expect, at the very best, to come out of this with a colostomy.

As I scrawled a hopeless attempt at a signature on the form, I was convinced it would be the last thing I would ever do – events were clearly cascading out of control and I had no confidence that anyone knew what they were doing. I had three thoughts as I calmly waited for the anesthetic to be pumped into my arm. Firstly, I quickly reviewed in my mind our financial position and concluded that I had not left Audrey and Georgina as secure as I would have liked – strike one. Secondly, I felt like I had not achieved everything in life I would have liked, with a strong sense of there being unfinished business – strike two. And thirdly, I was annoyed with myself for having signed up for a course of action that had left me open to what had always been my biggest fear: unplanned emergency surgery by a general surgeon who was unknown to me, as opposed to a Crohn's specialist who I had been able to research – strike three. I was not, I told myself, going out in a blaze of glory.

I was not panicky or tearful – that would come later – and I accepted that the end was inevitable. I can confirm that there is no bright light at the end of a passage; no welcoming Morgan Freeman-style voice; no gang of long-dead relatives beckoning me towards them or, indeed, urgently sending me back; no seventy-seven virgins and no hovering up around the ceiling watching my last minutes. Nothing. As I felt the anesthetic-induced blackness swimming into my brain, I had no doubt I was checking out permanently from the hotel of life.

No one was more surprised than me to find myself regaining consciousness, and who should be the first people I see in a life I thought had ended for sure? My wonderful wife and daughter; both smiling and looking extremely relieved, having been brought in by our good friend Gregg. As I came to, I heard their side of the story.

Audrey told me about her early morning call, the response to which had scared her rigid. Not long afterwards, a doctor had phoned her back to say I was gravely ill and she should come in immediately.

She then had to break this news to Georgina who reassured her mom that I was strong (I never knew that she thought this) and that I would be OK. Needless to say, despite their confidence in my constitution, it was a very long journey for them until, when nearing the hospital, Audrey received a second call saying that the surgery had gone well and I was going to be OK. Audrey also informed me that, on the previous day when the initial procedure had gone wrong, she had called my mother who had already jumped on a plane and would be arriving later that day.

After giving me this update, they were asked to leave me to rest and went off to the visitors' room. Even before they were out of the door, I had an overwhelming need to stick my hand under my surgical gown and search for the inevitable colostomy bag. I went down the left side first – nothing there! Maybe I was going to be doubly lucky: still alive and bag-free. As I moved my hand across to check the right-hand side, its progress was stopped by a completely unexpected obstruction in the middle. About the size of a grapefruit and a bit sponge-like in nature, I had no idea what this was until the thought flashed through my mind, "surely that can't be my scrotum?" It was indeed my scrotum but at least five times life-size.

The mystery was soon resolved as one of the first things Audrey said when they had come back in was, did I realize that my face and neck were completely swollen up? No, I didn't, but it seemed reasonable to assume that whatever had caused that had also had a similar inflationary effect on my kahunas. A passing doctor explained that the medics had pumped so much fluid into my system to try and restore some kind of circulation that it was far beyond the capacity of my kidneys to cope, so the body had stored it wherever it could.

The surgeon who had conducted this life-saving operation (a different surgeon to the one from the night before) stopped by and gave us all an update. Although my condition had been extremely grave, it had turned out to be a simple operation. After opening me up and pumping almost three liters of blood from my abdomen (half the body's total supply!), he had found an artery happily spurting away, so had quickly tied it off and then checked round everything else. There was no reason I shouldn't make a complete recovery in the fullness of time. There then followed a bed-side debate between another set of doctors as to whether or not I should be sent into the intensive care unit as the first stage of that process, the consensus being that I probably shouldn't, but it seemed a close-run decision.

As if all this had not been enough to endure, a few days later there happened another event that finally made me blow my stack. When it became apparent that my digestive system was rumbling back into life, the protocol was to outfit me in an adult-sized diaper as one could never tell what was going to come out while the system was cranking itself up again. However, I soon tired of that and, having taken it off, gave myself the challenge of conducting a mini bed-bath in the rear department to freshen things up. Much to my shock, I could feel something poking out that, if I didn't know better, felt like the end of a tube. What had gone wrong this time??? What did they leave in there????

I immediately pressed the emergency button to summon the nurse and ask her did I need to have this tube removed. "What tube?" was her less than encouraging response, "I'd better call the doctor." There then followed a similar debate when one of the junior doctors turned up. No, she didn't know what it was and therefore did not feel qualified to remove it in case it was something important. She would pass the problem up the line and page her boss to come and decide, but he was busy in theatre right now. Probably in a comedy, thought I.

My faith in doctors could not have sunk any lower after the two botched procedures, but it now plunged off the chart. I was livid. What if there was something else up there? Was it safe to move, or even breathe?

"Look," said I, "This tube is coming out in ten minutes whether your boss is here or not."

"Oh, he will be."

Needless to say, he wasn't, so I gingerly maneuvered the tube a fraction of an inch at a time until it finally emerged, some six inches long and about a quarter of an inch wide. When the head banana finally showed up, he was as mystified as the rest of us.

I'll be honest," he said, "I have no idea what this is or why it was here, but I will find out."

Much to his credit and my amazement, he did find out; in fact, he seemed to rattle quite a few cages in doing so. It transpired that the tube was the front end of the kind of suction tube dentists put in your mouth while they drill away. It had been part-inserted in me immediately after the double balloon endoscopy to help the passage of gas that had been pumped in during the procedure. Some enterprising staff member had fashioned the item from a leftover dentist's kit. While I had been moved up and down the bed having the X-rays done, it must have been pushed all the way in and had remained there through two major operations and several days of recovery. What a fiasco!

The next morning I was visited by a phalanx of medics and hospital administrators to explain themselves. But before they could do that, they had to listen to me.

"Firstly, a world-famous gastroenterologist punctures my bowel in front of three hundred expert witnesses and nobody notices a thing. Secondly, a surgeon leaves an artery bleeding in my gut; thirdly, nobody notices I am bleeding to death until the very last minute, and fourthly, random bits of plastic tube get shoved up my asshole and then completely forgotten about. Had I missed anything or was that a fair summary of my stay under their care?"

Needless to say there was lots of beard-pulling, eyeglass twiddling, shoe shuffling and not much in the way of a rebuttal. Case closed, Your Honor!

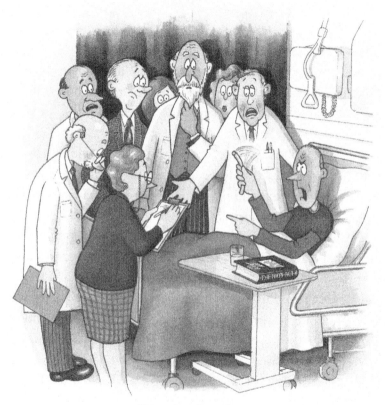

Doctoring the evidence

However, over the next couple of days they regrouped their forces and launched a counter-offensive. Had it not been pointed out to me that bowel perforation was a known complication of the enteroscopy? OK, I gave them that one, but if I had known that three hundred experts could not recognize when it happened before their eyes on live TV, I might have reconsidered my decision to go ahead. After that early fight-back, their case went rapidly downhill. The surgeon was ushered forward to claim that I was not bleeding when she sewed me up and that arteries could sometimes go into spasm when cut and not commence bleeding until hours later. Well, it had never happened to me before, and my mother, who had by now arrived to bolster my defenses, had been an operating theatre nurse for two years and never heard of it happening once.

On the third point as to why hadn't the bleeding been detected until I was through the pearly gates and disappearing up St. Peter's garden path, there was a difference of opinion. My mother had pored over my bedside notes and seen a slight drop in my blood pressure accompanied by a rise in my pulse taken at around 2am, some four hours after the surgery had finished. This, in her opinion, was a clear warning sign that should have prompted further measurements every fifteen minutes. However, I had not been checked again until 6am when, with me all but dead, the panic button had been pressed.

Their response was that once every four hours was the norm for stable patients, which I had been to that point. My mother vehemently disagreed with this but to no avail; they would not move and admit that a major error had been made and that it had been negligent to not check my vitals more frequently. To be fair to the night nurse, once she had realized something was wrong she had done everything right in immediately summoning the surgical team when every minute counted.

When it came to the tube-up-butt incident, they threw themselves on the mercy of the court. No excuses. It was a non-standard piece of equipment and its use hadn't been recorded, so its absence was not noticed in all the hullabaloo. They had already ordered that the box of dental off-cuts be thrown out and replaced by proper tubes fit for purpose and instituted a recording system for when one was put in and when removed. This list would be checked before patients were moved away from the endoscopy unit. Quite an impressive response, really, so I found it hard to stay angry about that part. However, I was still a bit peeved they had nearly killed me, even though I was not one to normally bear a grudge.

I then decided that all the stress of shouting at apologetic pen-pushers was doing me more harm than good, so I let them off the hook and settled back into my normal hospital routine of doing crosswords, watching DVD's, having morphine-induced bouts of terror and reporting on my fart count. As soon as I was out though, I got straight onto a firm of medical malpractice lawyers to see if I could seek redress. The outcome of my free hour's time with the ambulance-chaser was that, since I had survived, wasn't going to need round-the-clock nursing and couldn't point to a massive loss of income (all of which he sounded very disappointed to hear) I had no case to make. In Canada, your only hope is if you can point to such life-altering, or indeed life-ending, outcomes. But even when you have a rock-solid case, it takes years and costs you every penny you own in procuring expert witnesses, so I decided to let it lie.

The post-operative match report, later sent to me by the first surgeon, detailed that the rupture of the bowel had occurred between the two strictures so she had decided to take a sizeable chunk out as the surrounding bowel, including the two strictures, looked worse than useless anyway. I was now left with about five feet of small bowel from an original starting length, before I became ill thirty years previously, of approximately twenty feet – so I was down to a quarter of what nature had deemed sufficient for the job. Amazingly, this did not necessarily mean I would have short bowel syndrome as that usually only kicked in when you got down to your last three feet, but clearly there was not much room left for any more reductions.

My recovery went well, especially as I didn't have to worry about returning to work. Well before all this happened, I had decided to try my hand at becoming an author and had finished up the text of my first book – a history of Cadbury's – before the endoscopy procedure "just in case", which had turned out to be a very wise precaution indeed. I was soon feeling better than I had done for years and, without those troublesome and relatively ancient strictures, could begin planning on what would hopefully be a prolonged period of good health. The only outstanding issue was that I had to find a new hospital and gastroenterologist as, if I couldn't sue, at least I could take my business elsewhere.

Tip #99: It's More Important to be With the Best Surgeon Rather Than the Best Specialist

The best medical location for the ongoing maintenance of your condition, i.e. the domain of the specialist physician, may not be the best location for the surgical resolution of any complications that arise. Of course your goal is to be treated in a place where both physician and surgeon are top-notch experts in your condition, but what do you do when that cannot be achieved? My advice is to go with the best surgeon – the wrong surgeon can kill you a lot easier than can the wrong physician.

Once I was home and mobile again, I huddled with my family doctor, who had been appalled at the sequence of events that had taken place, to plot the way forwards. If I had not gone to her suggesting a change of care regime, I have no doubt she would have insisted anyway. It turned out there were a couple of Toronto hospitals which conducted far more Crohn's surgeries than the place I had been, so how to choose between them?

Here's where I relied on information I had picked up at CCFC meetings. There are differences in the incidence of Crohn's disease between different countries and different races – nobody really knows why. Canada has one of the highest rates in the world as do Jewish people, so when I saw that one of her two recommended hospitals was Toronto's Mount Sinai, famous in the city for its many and generous Jewish benefactors, my thinking was this should be the busiest hospital in the world for Crohn's disease. Perhaps not quite, but I did my internet research and the set-up looked far closer to my first hospital in Birmingham in having a specialized Crohn's facility with dedicated surgical teams and plenty of ongoing research programs.

So, once again, she arranged for my transfer and that is where I have been cared for, incident-free, ever since. My new gastroenterologist is of the view that, since I do not have too much bowel left, it is better to keep a more vigilant eye on the state of what remains through a more proactive program of imaging. However, when he suggested a barium meal, I flatly rejected the idea. I just did not want to risk any more radiation.

"OK," he said, "In that case there are some new options we can try."

Technology marches on.

In early 2010 I underwent an abdominal ultrasound scan, a small bowel MRI, a colonoscopy and a gastroscopy, so he had two views of my insides and a view from both the top and bottom end. Pretty thorough, if you ask me. And the good news from all this eyeballing was that, for the first time in my adult life, there was no sign of strictures or any active Crohn's disease at all. The final surgery, although mega-traumatic, had removed all my previously diseased bowel and the Infliximab had indeed turned out to be a miracle drug, preventing any active inflammation arising.

Will it last forever? Probably not. But then, given everything that has happened to me in the past, I could never have anticipated feeling this good, so who knows?

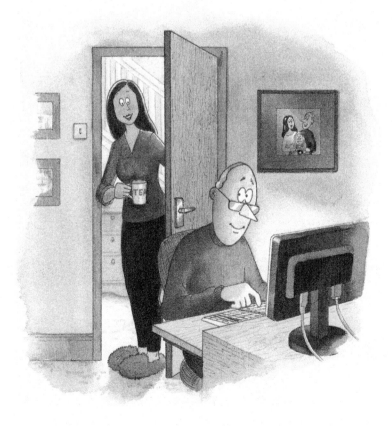

Looking Forward

A Short History of Medicine:
2000 B.C. – "Here, eat this root."
1000 A.D. – "That root is heathen; say this prayer."
1850 A.D. – "That prayer is superstition; drink this potion."
1940 A.D. – "That potion is snake oil; swallow this pill."
1985 A.D. – "That pill is ineffective; take this antibiotic."
2000 A.D. – "That antibiotic is artificial. Here, eat this root."

– Anon

WHILE I DO not consider myself a medical expert, I am undoubtedly a veteran patient. During the past thirty-four years, since my first real symptom scared me to death in the john of a student residence, I have undergone thirteen surgeries (seven major and six minor), three of which were within the same twenty-four hours; had well over a hundred consultations with gastroenterologists; had at least two hundred blood tests; taken at least a dozen different drugs, often for years at a time; been irradiated to the Chernobyl standards; lost five-sixths of my small bowel, and had half a dozen complete strangers stick their index fingers up my butt. And I have never been happier.

I often hear people say things like, "At least I have got my health" or "Good health is everything." No it isn't – that's just something healthy people say before they get ill. I haven't had good health since I was a teenager and I do not feel that I have lost, or been denied, "everything". Far from it. I consider myself to have had a marvelous life so far and in no way feel short-changed.

Tip #100: Illness is Not an Aberration, It's Part of Life

Complaining about being ill is like a broken pencil - pointless. Crohn's was in my genes and I have had it for almost two-thirds of my life. Having Crohn's is a part of who I am. How I chose to deal with it has, in a large part, made me the person I am today, so what have I got to complain about really?

If I had to put my finger on the biggest single reason I feel this way, it is because I have always believed that one has to take ownership for the management of illness; that way I still feel I have ownership for the direction of my life. Once you give ownership over to the medical profession, you are signing away having any sort of control over the rest of your life. There are many fine doctors out there, but it is a mistake to assume they are qualified to run your life for you.

Crohn's disease was first identified over seventy years ago, so you would think it should be well understood by now. Especially when you consider that I have had the illness for over thirty years with a very well documented case history. Yet not one doctor on this planet can tell me what will happen next - hardly the basis for handing over the planning of my life. Taking ownership for the course of your life, including the highly unpredictable illness part of it, is the key to making the most of the hand life has dealt you.

Tip #101: Don't Look Back

Being ill is indeed a drawback if you spend all your time and energy looking back, thinking what life would have been like without illness. But when life with illness is spent

looking forward, thinking about and preparing for the possibilities that life holds within the limits that your illness im-
poses, it is no drawback at all, it is just part of your life. (So
says the man who has just spent five months looking back
and documenting his illness!)

I hope that in my relating to you these events, you are able to gain
some benefit as you navigate your own path through Crohn's
disease and the medical system. I have not found this to be a
cathartic experience, in fact quite the opposite, but if even just one
tip is of value to you, then I am glad that I did it.

Postscript: While all the events in this book are true, the names
of the doctors and hospitals have been changed.

About the Author

DIAGNOSED WITH Crohn's disease at the age of 25 in 1983 after seven years of increasingly dire symptoms, John Bradley spent the next 27 years battling the illness, relapses, symptoms, the medical system, drugs, side effects, surgeries and doctors while finding the time to build a career, marry and become a father. He is now a full-time author and lives near Toronto.

CPSIA information can be obtained
at www.ICGtesting.com
Printed in the USA
LVOW03s0645251117
557523LV00011B/1123/P